THE FACTS

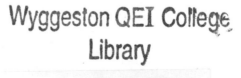

THE FACTS FROM OXFORD UNIVERSITY PRESS

Ageing: the facts
(second edition) Nicholas Coni, William Davison, and Stephen Webster

Alcoholism: the facts
(third edition) Donald W. Goodwin

Arthritis and rheumatism:
the facts (second edition) J. T. Scott

Asthma: the facts
(third edition) Donald J. Lane

Autism: the facts
Simon Baron-Cohen and Patrick Bolton

Back pain: the facts
(third edition) Malcolm I. V. Jayson

Bowel cancer: the facts
John M. A. Northover and Joel D. Kettner

Cancer: the facts
(second edition) Michael Whitehouse and Maurice Slevin

Childhood leukaemia: the facts
John S. Lilleyman

Contraception: the facts
(second edition) Peter Bromwich and Tony Parsons

Coronary heart disease:
the facts (second edition)
Desmond Julian and Claire Marley

Cystic fibrosis: the facts
(third edition) Ann Harris and Maurice Super

Dyslexia and other learning difficulties:
the facts
Mark Selikowitz

Eating disorders: the facts
(third edition) Suzanne Abraham and Derek Llewellyn-Jones

Eczema in childhood: the facts
David J. Atherton

Epilepsy: the facts
(second edition) Anthony Hopkins and Richard Appleton

Head injury: the facts
Dorothy Gronwall, Philip Wrightson and Peter Waddell

Healthy skin: the facts
Rona M. MacKie

Liver disease and gallstones: the facts
(second edition) Alan G. Johnson and David R. Triger

Lung cancer: the facts
(second edition) Chris Williams

Migraine: the facts
(second edition) J. N. Blau

Miscarriage: the facts
(second edition) Gillian C. L. Lachelin

Multiple sclerosis: the facts
(third edition) Bryan Matthews

Muscular dystrophy: the facts
Alan E. H. Emery

Obsessive–compulsive disorder:
the facts
Padmal de Silva and Stanley Rachman

Panic disorder: the facts
Padmal de Silva and Stnaley Rachman

Thyroid disease: the facts
(second edition) R. I. S. Bayliss and W. M. G. Tunbridge

ALSO FROM OXFORD
UNIVERSITY PRESS

Breast cancer: a guide for every woman
Michael Baum, Christobel Saunders, and Sheena Meredith

Fighting for life
Gilbert Park and Kieron Saunders

Forbidden drugs: understanding drugs and why people take them
Philip Robson

Friendly fire: explaining autoimmune disease
David Isenberg and John Morrow

Unplanned pregnancy: your choices
Ann Furedi

Cancer

THE FACTS
Second Edition

• •

By

MICHAEL WHITEHOUSE

Director, CRC Wessex Medical Oncology Unit, Southampton

and

MAURICE SLEVIN

Consultant Medical Oncologist, St Bartholomew's Hospital London

Oxford   New York   Tokyo
OXFORD UNIVERSITY PRESS
1996

Oxford University Press, Walton Street, Oxford OX2 6DP

Oxford   New York
Athens   Auckland   Bangkok   Bombay
Calcutta   Cape Town   Dar es Salaam   Delhi
Florence   Hong Kong   Istanbul   Karachi
Kuala Lumpur   Madras   Madrid   Melbourne
Mexico City   Nairobi   Paris   Singapore
Taipei   Tokyo   Toronto

and associated companies in
Berlin   Ibadan

Oxford is a trade mark of Oxford University Press

Published in the United States
by Oxford University Press Inc., New York

A catalogue record for this book is available from the British Library
(Data available)

Library of Congress Cataloging in Publication Data

ISBN 0 19 261695 1

Typeset by Palimpsest Book Production Limited,
Polmont, Stirlingshire
Printed in Great Britain on acid-free paper by
Biddles Ltd, Guildford and King's Lynn

Preface

Those who spend their working lives looking after people with cancer know only too well that the most rational individual is thrown into turmoil when told that their illness is caused by cancer. Suddenly any of the apparent certainties in life are thrown into disarray. There is a sense of loss of control, of being unable to influence one's own life, a complete uncertainty of what the future may hold and, inevitably, anxieties about what visits to hospital may entail. If that is not enough there is often a fear of dependence on others and the implications of what their own vulnerability may mean for their families.

'Cancer' when it is first voiced to someone newly diagnosed is interpreted as an overwhelming threat to life as they know it and with this realization they come face to face with their own mortality. In the maelstrom of emotions which come with being told of a cancer it is essential to begin to re-create some elements of security. This is particularly necessary since without such information there is a risk that imagination and pessimism combine to fuel feelings of despair. Although this initial reaction is for many people inappropriate these are often their first emotions on being told their diagnosis. It is only when the full facts of their condition are known that they begin to understand something of their illness and how they may play their part in containing its influence, thus regaining some sense of control of their life.

Cancer: the facts helps with this process by providing information which helps towards an understanding of different cancers, how they are caused (where this is known), how they may present, how they may be diagnosed, how they may be treated, and also gives some insight into the impact cancer may have on people's lives.

This book is intended not as an encyclopaedia but as a source of understandable information which may be helpful in putting cancer and its problems into perspective. It may be used by sufferers and their families to help understand particular situations and so to be able to ask the most relevant questions of carers. Although not comprehensive it is intended to give some idea of the current management policies for different cancers and the reasons why particular managements may be appropriate. Above all, it is intended to provide information which may help those who, for whatever reason, have some interest in cancer.

The authors would like to acknowledge the help of those who have contributed to the writing of this book. First and foremost are those whom they have cared for with cancer who, during the course of their professional lives, have taught them most of what is important in looking after people with cancer. They are particularly indebted to Senor Jose Carreras for giving his own inspirational view of living life despite cancer in the Foreword to this book; to Dr Jane Toms of the Cancer Research Campaign for reading the manuscript and helping with facts and figures; to Dr Tim Sheard for his chapter on complementary medicine; to Annie Jackson of BACUP, an expert on writing about cancer for patients and their families, for her invaluable help and advice, and for permission to reproduce some of the illustrations and information; to those of our patients who read the manuscripts in preparation and by their comments helped to improve the chapters and to our wives and our families who tolerated our time away from them while we worked on this book and whose encouragement sustained us throughout its preparation.

Southampton   M.W
London   M.S.
June 1996

Contents

Foreword by José Carreras ix
Introduction xi
1 What is cancer? 1
2 History 7
3 Some cancer statistics 14
4 Screening for cancer 21
5 How do cancers cause symptoms? 26
6 Tests for cancer and how cancer is investigated 33
7 Treatments for cancer 43
    Surgery 43
    Radiotherapy 46
    Chemotherapy 56
    Bone marrow and stem cell transplants 62
8 Cancers by site of origin 69
    Head and neck 69
    Salivary glands 72
    Eyes 74
    Thyroid 75
    Brain 78
    Lung 82
    Breast 88
    Ovary 100
    Cervix 105
    Uterus 112
    Oesophagus 116
    Stomach 120
    Bowel 126
    Pancreas 134
    Liver 140
    Adrenal 143

Cancer: the facts

	Kidney	146
	Bladder	149
	Prostate	151
	Urethra	155
	Penis	155
	Testis	155
	Bone	160
	Soft tissue	164
	Skin	167
	Lymphomas	173
	Myeloma	184
	Leukaemias	187
	Childhood cancers	195
9	Quality of life during cancer treatment	201
10	Living with advanced cancer	209
11	Complementary medicine in cancer care (by Dr Tim Sheard)	219
Useful addresses		231
Index		237

Foreword

José Carreras, President, International Leukaemia Foundation

• •

I deeply appreciate the authors' kind invitation to write the foreword to *Cancer: the facts*. It gives me the chance to be in contact with people to whom I would like to bring a message of hope.

Most likely you are reading this book because in one way or another, you are close to the disease. Let me first of all tell you the most important 'fact' of all: cancer can be beaten.

My modest contribution to the ambitious work of the authors comes from my own personal experience as a patient. Testimonies such as mine are frequent today. Thanks to the enormous progress achieved by researchers all over the world, more and more patients are winning the fight. I was fortunate enough to be among them.

However, science and medicine, while essential, are not enough. It takes a lot of courage from the patient and the loving support of family and those closest to overcome the threat posed by the disease.

Knowing what lies ahead at each moment is also an important source of encouragement. Many times, the prospects of an invasive therapy, or an aggressive treatment may be devastating. The directness of the doctor-patient relationship can sometimes bring difficult episodes in the course of the curative process. However, proper information, with no false expectations but, most important, no unjustified fears is a crucial element in helping patients and their families.

Nietzsche once wrote 'Calm the imagination of the patient so that at least he does not suffer more from his thoughts about the illness than from the illness itself'. I think that the authors have successfully contributed to this sympathetic purpose. Reading this book will doubtless bring decisive support to individuals needing to face illness with renewed courage.

Cancer: the facts

Finally, let me share with you what I recall as being the fundamental source of strength in my recovery: even if there is only a small chance of survival, that particular chance is yours and the one you fight for.

Jose Carreras

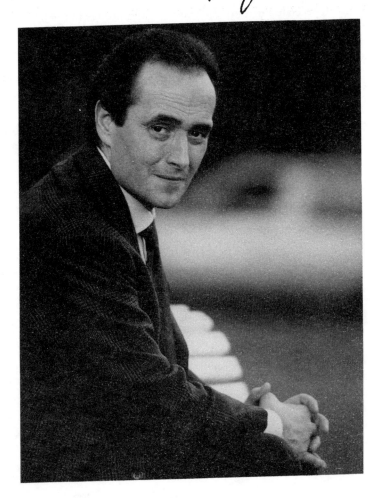

Introduction

· ·

You may remember that the White Rabbit, while trying to give evidence, was hardly helped by Alice during her journey through Wonderland. However the King of Hearts was more helpful when the White Rabbit appeared uncertain as to how to proceed. 'Begin at the beginning', the King said, very gravely, 'and go on till you come to the end: then stop'.

More than likely you will not want to read this book from beginning to end, but instead to return to various sections to build up your own understanding. You may come to it with a specific question,

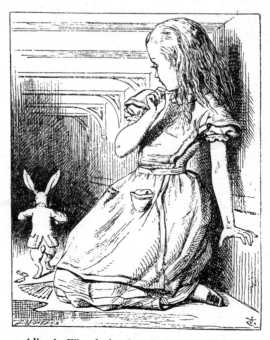

Alice in Wonderland and the White Rabbit.

or perhaps to gain a better general appreciation of a particular topic without necessarily wishing to follow the advice of the King. This is intended as a book for browsing, and also one where those with specific questions may find straightforward answers. There is no beginning to a story about cancer, and since our understanding about the cancer process, about its investigation, treatment, and the care of those who have it is constantly changing, there is no end.

It may seem curious that a word like 'cancer' can cause dread and yet few people really understand what it is. Perhaps it is feared just for this reason, for in the absence of knowledge it is possible to imagine all manner of horrors, and human nature ensures that many of us will do just that. In the past, mankind had greater terrors—famine, the plague, syphilis, tuberculosis, but as each has been contained so cancer, remaining unaffected by each advance, has gained in prominence.

We are not helped in our perspective of cancer by its immediate history in the twentieth century. It might have been thought that a disease process which Chapter 2 tells us is so old, would have by now had the proper appreciation in our folklore. Not so. The biology of cancer only began to be appreciated 200 years ago, and has been misunderstood regularly even as recently as the lifetime of most who read this book.

The healers, although promoting their art, have over the centuries tended to write about their failures, for good health draws little of the attention elicited by protracted illness. Rare success is readily forgotten when dominated by frequent failure. With each failure, comes the temptation to try a different remedy, and when this fails, so the appraisal of therapy becomes less realistic and the willingness to try even the bizarre is increased. But sound counsel is not something to reserve to the end; practical, accurate information can help cancer patients to play the leading role in managing their illnesses.

Today the surgeon can refashion tissues in a most remarkable way. He can often remove all visible evidence of the offending tumour. However many early twentieth century surgeons lost interest in the patients who were not cured, not because they were callow men, but because their skills could not help them to aid their patients. Many of us still remember surgical ward rounds where the sad figure of a patient with advanced cancer was often ignored. Is it any wonder that relatives on whom the burden of care fell, remember cancer as 'the terrible illness'? That mythology was perpetuated by the silence which would surround patients, because often they were not told their diagnosis.

Radiotherapy, a marvellous development early this century, offered new hope to those who had failed to be cured by the surgeon's knife. Although this new technology kindled interest and enthusiasm for treating cancer, the impact of this discovery does not compare with that of drugs which can act to control or eliminate a cancer. We have learned that we must think about cancers as a disorder which may affect different parts of the body. Surgery and radiotherapy may be very useful in dealing with the site where the cancer first begins, while drug treatment can influence cancer cells far outside the treated area. As you read this book you will begin to understand how various treatments may be used, and the thinking behind how they are chosen.

The person who benefits from surgery, radiotherapy, or drug treatment may pass virtually unnoticed, or at least with continuing good health, their problems are rapidly forgotten. Those who are less fortunate tend to impress more vividly. The symptoms of illness, the side-effects of treatment all contribute to the commonly held images associated with cancer. Some of these problems will remain, for illnesses of all kinds and can still elude the most modern medical skills, but cancer medicine is today the fastest changing area of modern medicine. The phenomenal progress of the last 50 years has only recently been shared with those for whom it is most relevant—the patients themselves. Today no one need ever feel that nothing can be done for them—there is *always* something that will be helpful in one way or another. Awareness of cancer is increasingly that it is a medical problem like any other. And, like any medical problem, we must define it, and then deal with it. Perhaps this may help to understand the difficult and frightening situations that arise when at first no treatment seems to be helpful.

When you browse through this book you may gain a better understanding of what cancer is, how it may arise, how it may behave, how different cancers may be influenced by surgery, radiotherapy, and drug therapy, and how cancer compares with other illnesses. The index may lead you to specific topics for a more detailed answer to your question. Whatever your motive for informing yourself, it is to be hoped that after doing so, you will not feel that 'cancer' is taboo, but something which may be talked about openly with relatives and friends. Cancer is after all a community problem—different perhaps from inflation, the moral dilemma surrounding nuclear weapons, or the problems facing education, but like them, requiring a solution to benefit us all.

Dedications

Mike Whitehouse
for:
Diane, Alex, Fiona, and Vanessa

Maurice Slevin
for:
My wife, Nicky, and my daughters,
Lindi, Amy, and Susannah

1   *What is cancer?*

It may seem curious how a word like cancer can cause dread, and yet few people really understand what cancer is. Perhaps this is one of the reasons why it is so feared, because in the absence of knowledge it is possible to imagine the worst and human nature means that most of us do just that. An incurable spreading ulcer, crab-like in shape, was given the Latin name cancer by the ancient Romans. Words used to describe cancers, such as 'tumour' or 'neoplasm' tell us little or nothing about what cancer really is. They are really descriptive—'tumour' meaning no more than a swelling, and 'neoplasm', literally 'new disease'. As mentioned in Chapter 2 a more recently coined term 'oncology' derived from the Greek 'onkos', a swelling, is applied to the part of medical science which relates to tumours. 'Carcinoma' is derived from the Greek for crab, but this term is now restricted to cancers of covering tissues such as skin and the lining of the mouth and intestine, and another word 'sarcoma' is used for cancers of supporting tissues such as bone, fat, muscle, and connecting tissues. Clearly no help in understanding cancer is to come from examining these terms more closely.

To do so we really need to go back to how we ourselves are formed, for one of the fastest growing tumours is the human foetus. It is perhaps unfair to compare this with a cancer, for the foetus is an example of normal growth, but there are many lessons to be learned from looking at the normal in order to help us better understand in what way cancer is different. Each one of us is made up of some fifteen million million cells, but we all start life at the moment of conception from the equivalent of one cell. The cell is the basic unit of life and some living organisms consist of one cell only, but even in these, it is a highly complex structure. Cancer too starts from one cell, and like the first cell of the foetus seems to be invested with a fantastic potential for growth, but before we look at the cancer cell, let us look at the way we ourselves develop from one cell.

Once the ovum of the mother is fertilized by the sperm of the father, this allows a remarkable genetic material from each parent called DNA, which can carry an enormous amount of information, to combine within the nucleus of a newly formed single cell. This then begins to divide forming new cells. Each of these can also divide to form new cells, each one containing the same genetic material carrying characteristics derived from each parent. This process continues almost hour by hour, each cell giving rise to a fantastic hierarchy of cells. It can well be imagined that some quite remarkable controlling mechanisms are necessary to fashion just one tiny part of a baby. During early development, cells with different tasks migrate in the forming body to the correct location, and there organize themselves in relationship to one another, and to cells around them to form different structures. Different cells join others of a similar kind to form tissues—the skin is the most obvious example, but even in skin there are different cells, as for example the cells around hairs, on the lips, the inside of the mouth, and beneath the eyelid. The blink of an eyelid reveals structures and mechanisms which man strives to mimic with all the modern skills of engineering and electronics at his disposal, but the result is only the poorest compromise. This is all to say that in nature growth and development happen in a controlled and harmonized way, which is still impossible to reproduce artificially. It is from an individual cell, within such a tissue, that a cancer may arise. What is quite remarkable, when one considers the numbers of cells involved, is not that cancer occurs, but that it does so infrequently.

Mammalian cells, that is cells from warm blooded animals, are very similar in structure. Each has an outer skin called the cell membrane and a central nucleus. Between the nucleus and the cell membrane is a jelly like material called 'cytoplasm'. Just as the outer covering including the skin of various mammals differs depending on the environment in which they live, i.e. polar bears, monkeys, whales, and man, so the cell membrane has different structures depending on where it is to be, and what function it has. To give an example, the cells of the skin must stick to one another all the time—if they and cells of some other structures did not, we would literally fall apart. On the other hand, blood cells cannot stick together if they are to circulate in blood vessels. In addition, they have different functions and so their cell membranes have some features not found in skin cells, and in particular they lack the structures that attach cells to one another. In the centre of the cell is its brain—the nucleus. Here messages are received and instructions sent to different parts of the cell. Within each nucleus is a very long piece of DNA which is coiled and folded to fit within the nucleus. Just before a cell divides the genes, each of which determines the characteristics of the cell, are packaged into chromosomes so that they can pass from one dividing cell to the new daughter cells. The cell behaviour is, quite literally, governed from the nucleus. It may give the instruction to manufacture substances, or equally may receive a message. When a substance of a particular shape binds to a 'receptor' on the cell membrane into which it fits perfectly, this causes a message to be sent to the nucleus, equally a chemical can come into the cell and have a similar effect. An example of the result of such messages is that the cell can be prompted to multiply. This happens when skin is damaged; the chemicals which are released from the damaged cells trigger repair mechanisms to become active in surrounding cells and new cells are produced to cover the damaged area.

In between the nucleus and the cell membrane is the cytoplasm. This contains the skeleton of the cell which stops it collapsing, and may in certain cases, help it to move. In our own bodies, the cell contains its own energy production and storage systems necessary for the cell to live. In addition, since cells of various tissues have different functions the special characteristics associated with different functions are found in the cytoplasm and in the cell membrane.

In the body most cells are in a steady 'resting' state and in normal circumstances this is only changed when tissues are injured. However a few tissues are constantly repairing themselves, for example the bowel and skin. Others are constantly active such as hair follicle cells, or constantly dividing to produce new daughter cells as happens in the ovaries, the testes, and the bone marrow. The rate of activity varies from tissue to tissue and in one, the uterus, it is cyclical, a new stage of repair occurring after menstruation. Throughout the body these are orderly processes but when they become less orderly well recognized illnesses which are quite unassociated with cancer may occur. A good example is 'psoriasis'—a disorder where overproduction of cells occurs in localized areas of skin.

For cancers to occur several things must happen but in particular the orderly behaviour of the cell must be lost. Unlike the cell repairing a wound, which stops dividing when the process is complete, the cancer cell ignores messages to stop dividing. It is almost as though the cell was set to 'automatic'. The mechanisms involved are gradually becoming better understood. In some cases a 'gene' (the genetic switch controlling cell multiplication—formed by a unique piece of DNA) becomes switched on either because it is directly modified or because another gene nearby makes it more active. Alternatively a gene may be lost which would otherwise have inhibited the 'active' gene. In extremely rare cancers such as retinoblastoma, occurring in the eyes of very young children, this last mechanism is recognized, but generally the cause of a particular cancer is unknown. Some risk factors are known. The scrotal cancers mentioned in Chapter 2 are caused by cancer-causing chemicals in soot, so called carcinogens; these react directly with the DNA of the cells and they actually cause a change in the genetic material called a 'mutation'. Very rarely this may result in a cancer. There are a number of chemicals such as benzene which are known to increase the risk of cancer. Another example is napthalene dyes which are now strictly controlled but became recognized as a cause of bladder cancer. Asbestos, which is produced from a naturally occurring mineral, was for many years used as a heat-insulating material. This may cause a cancer of the lining of the lungs many years after exposure to the dust. The best known risk from a common source of carcinogens is tobacco smoke. This contains minute quantities of a chemical, 3,4 benzpyrene, which at higher concentrations will regularly produce skin cancers if painted onto the skin of mice. Apart from tobacco smoke the use of known carcinogens is strictly controlled by legislation. Exposure to radiation may also in certain circumstances produce 'mutations' (changes in the genetic message) which lead to an increased risk of cancers. The best known example of this is the small but definite increase in cancer seen amongst the survivors of atomic bombing in the Second World War. Ultraviolet radiation (particularly apparent in strong sunlight) exposure, if prolonged, has a similar effect. It is well known that exposure to intense sunlight over the years may cause an increase in certain skin cancers, in particular 'basal cell' cancer, 'squamous cell' cancer, and 'malignant melanoma'.

The precise role of viruses in causing cancer is as yet unknown. Simple infection is clearly not enough to start the process for otherwise cancers would be much more common in younger age groups. It does seem that a complex interaction between viruses and other conditions such as environmental carcinogens or genetic defects is required to trigger the development of a cancer and even then that it would only rarely be successful. The Epstein–Barr virus (EBV), which is present throughout the world, has been implicated in a cancer of lymph gland tissue in Africa—Burkitt's lymphoma. A consequence of the AIDS virus infection is an impaired immune resistance which seems to permit a rare tumour to develop in the skin and other tissues—Kaposi's sarcoma. A relatively common virus, the human papilloma virus (HPV), is now thought to play a part in causing cancer of the cervix (see p.42).

Certain environmental factors are undoubtedly important, for example chemicals within the diet are a focus of much interest. Some important questions are likely to be answered by current research into why it is that the Japanese have a much higher incidence of stomach cancer and a much lower incidence of bowel cancer than are found in the USA. Despite this, Japanese who have lived their lives in the USA lose this trait and become like their American counterparts, having a much higher incidence of bowel cancer than their relatives in Japan. These effects only occur after many many years so that short-term changes in diet cannot be expected either to increase or decrease the risk of developing bowel cancer and will certainly not influence its behaviour once it has occurred.

It is probable that before the cancer begins the affected tissues become rather less stable. Pathologists are familiar with this state which may in some cases be called 'pre-cancerous'. They see cells and tissues taken for biopsy which look less orderly than is normal and when individual cells are examined these show irregularities in the appearance of the nucleus and its surrounding cytoplasm. When a cell becomes malignant very little may be apparent for some considerable time. After all, many millions of cells are required to form a lump the size of a pea. Little by little a clump of cells forms until eventually a nodule which can actually be felt is formed. The rate at which this grows depends on many things but it is possible that some tumours take weeks to grow to a detectable size while others may take years. Of course the leukaemias which are diseases of the blood-forming tissue in the bone marrow rarely form lumps but they do tend to crowd out the normal cells and the disease becomes apparent because of this (see p.187). The main features of solid cancers are the mechanical problems caused by their growth and the secondary lumps caused by cells breaking off from the main tumour and spreading to other parts of the body via the blood, lymph, or even by direct extension. These secondary clumps of cancer cells are called 'metastases'.

These metastases, and indeed the primary may grow within a vital organ and eventually compromise its function. Rarely, cancers actually produce large quantities of certain chemical substances in quantity which at normal levels are important for the body's function, but which in high concentration may produce disturbing effects. Certain substances secreted by cancers can cause very general symptoms such as weakness, anaemia, depression, constipation, night sweats, and other fairly commonplace symptoms. Effective treatment of the cancer will control these problems. It is the improved understanding of the cancer process and of the behaviour of the cancer cell which has so improved the prospects for the patient with cancer.

2 History

· ·

At the far end of a long peninsula, in south-west Turkey, is the ancient citadel of Knidos. Here was once a thriving community of 60 000 people, living among temples, theatres, roads, and all manner of buildings of extraordinary sophistication. Today, these remnants of Byzantine and Greek civilization litter the hillside now foraged by goats and cattle. A handful of peasants eke out a living from passing boats and a small military out-post guards with civility this footprint of one of the greatest civilizations in the history of man. Looking to the north-west from this barren hillside over bleached rocks and beyond the pastel blue of the now silted harbour, across a mere 10 miles of open sea, lies the landmass of the island of Kos. Here, around 450 BC before Knidos had reached its prime, a man was born who was to lay the foundations of modern medicine—Hippocrates. In later life Hippocrates, who combined observation with perceptive interpretation, wrote a series of remarkable treatises, which enable us to gain some knowledge of the illnesses of the time. Among his writings is a treatise entitled '*On Carcinosis*'. In this is a description of what appears to be cancer of the breast: 'a woman from Abdera developed carcinoma of the breast, and through the nipple there was sero-sanguinous discharge, when the discharge ceased, she died'. The term 'carcinoma' is now used to describe cancers which arise in covering tissues, the suffix 'oma' meaning swelling. Hippocrates also used the term 'onkos' to describe a swelling, and although he probably did not intend this exclusively to describe cancer, from it has come the word 'oncology' which literally means the study of swellings, but which today is used to describe all cancer-related disciplines.

Two thousand years before the microscope was invented, the diagnosis of cancer depended on a combination of experienced observation and guesswork, for there was no means of proving the fact. Some infections can mimic cancers and would certainly have caused confusion. However Hippocrates obviously felt secure in identifying a group of conditions as cancers, so much so that he wrote about their treatment:

'It is better not to apply any treatment in cases of occult cancer, for, if treated, the patients die quickly; but if not treated, they survive for a long time' (Hippocrates, *Aphorism No. 38*).

At about the time of Hippocrates, Atossa the wife of Darius, had a massive ulcerating cancer of the breast which she concealed for many years. This prompted Herodotus to write (430 BC) of her foolishness and to advance the concept of early detection and treatment. One can understand that she should keep quiet for elsewhere can be found reference to the treatment of breast cancers with a 'fire-drill'—probably some form of cautery but almost certainly as fearsome as it sounds.

There are few medical writings before Hippocrates, however the papyrus writings of the Egyptians as far back as 3000 BC do contain some clues. One of the best known—the Edwin Smith Surgical Papyrus Case 45—is translated as follows. 'If thou examinest a man having bulging tumours on his breast, (and) thou findest that swellings have spread over his breasts; if thou puttest thy hand upon his breast, upon more tumours, (and) thou findest them very cool, there being no fever at all therein, when thy hand touches him; they have no granulation, they form no fluid, they do not generate secretions of fluid, and they are not bulging to thy hand. . . . . Swellings on his breast are large, spreading and hard; touching them is like touching a ball of wrappings; the comparision is to a green haemat fruit, which is hard and cool under thy hand, like touching those swellings which are on his breast.' This may well have been a cancer, but it seems likely since life expectancy was short and that cancer becomes commoner with increasing age that cancers would have been uncommon.

Egyptian art shows various 'tumours' such as a hydrocoele, hernias, and enlargement of the male breast, but no obvious cancer.

The Egyptians of antiquity did preserve some internal organs and at least one mummy probably had cancer of the ovary. Most other evidence of early cancers has had to come from examining the remains of skeletons—several have been found, particularly in the skull. The earliest example is that found in the backbone of a dinosaur!

Cancer is therefore not a new disease, but a very old one, and although ill understood, was recorded with increasing frequency with the passage of the centuries. In the second century AD another physician of stature, Galen, noted that the distension caused by tumours was similar to that of a swollen animal. He wrote 'Carcinoma is a tumour, malignant and indurated, ulcerated or non-ulcerated. It is named after the animal cancer. . . . . . And on the breasts we often saw tumours resembling exactly the animal cancer, and just as the animal's legs are on either side of its body, so do the veins stretched by the unnatural tumour resemble (the animal) cancer in shape'. Like Hippocrates he preached against intervention when the disease was advanced, but lent some justification to the idea of screening even then by concluding that early disease could be cured: 'and the early cancer we have cured, but the one that rose to considerable size without surgery, nobody has cured'. Description of illness would have been something of a luxury, and most healers would have given their energies to treatment, so that only sporadic reports of cancer occur in early medical history. Hippocrates did recognize cancer of the uterus, but it was not until the sixth century that Aetios of Amida described a similar case. A famous Saxon surgeon, John of Ardern, described cancer of the rectum in the fourteenth century, and in 1700, Gendron published a book entitled *'Causative Hypotheses'* in which, like Hippocrates, he noted that only localized lesions could be cured.

Early science tended to depend upon visual observation but Paracelsus tried to use some of the ideas of alchemy to gain a better understanding of disease. He advocated a search for the essence of disease through combustion. After examining burnt tissues he decided that cancer was due to an excess of mineral salts in the blood. This idea was contested by Astruc of Montpellier who after comparing incinerated breast cancer with burnt beef steak, decided that it was no more salty. Despite such uncomfortable theorizing the nature of cancer was poorly understood, but Le Dran (1685–1770) developed the idea that cancer may start as a local tumour and then spread elsewhere via lymph (the fluid which contains essential fluids from blood which surrounds tissues and cells). When cancer does spread to form a separate island of cancer remote from the initial focus it is called a metastasis. Recamier (1774–1852) first described this process.

It was not until the early days of the post-mortem (literally examination 'after death') that cancers of different organs were documented. European culture and academia were on the ascendancy by the early eighteenth century, spawning scholars in every discipline. Among these, was the first great pathologist Morgagni, who in 1761 published a text describing cancers occurring in different internal organs including the lung, oesophagus, stomach, rectum, and uterus. Other classical descriptions were to follow, but it was

Percival Pott in 1775 who recognized a possible causative factor
for some cancers in his description of cancer of the scrotum in
chimney sweeps. In these unfortunates, it was the cancer-inducing
activity of the chemicals in the soot which was recognized to cause
the cancer. This might well be described as the first recognized
environmental cause of a cancer. Later other possible associations
were noted such as that between smoking and cancer of the lip
and nose. Life expectancy was still low, but in the search for
information which characterized 'The Age of Reason' meticulous
documentation led to the recognition of various cancers. Despite
these remarkable observations the true nature of cancer was still
not related to cells, but in 1838 Johannes Mueller made this vital
association.

At last some rationale could be applied to therapy, but as many
early case reports reveal, ideas of treatment were neither original nor
effective. The description of a case of leukaemia by John Hughes
Bennett in 1845 gives some insight into approaches to treatment nearly
150 years ago.

• •

'John Menteith, age 28, a slater, married, admitted into the clinical ward of
the Royal Infirmary, February 28, 1845. He is of dark complexion, usually
healthy and temperate, states that twenty months ago he was affected with
great listlessness on exertion, which has continued to this time. In June last he
noticed a tumour on the left side of the abdomen, which has gradually increased
in size till four months since when it became stationary.

It was never painful till last week, after the application of three blisters to it;
since then several other small tumours have appeared in his neck, axillae, and
groins, at first attended with a sharp pain, which has now, however, disappeared
from all of them. Before he noticed the tumour he had frequently vomited in
the morning. The bowels are usually constipated, appetite good, is not subject
to indigestion, has had no vomiting since he noticed the tumour. He used
chiefly purgative medicines, especially croton oil, has employed friction with
a liniment, and had the tumour blistered.

At present there appears a large tumour, extending from the ribs to the groin,
and from the spinal column to the umbilicus, lying on the left side. It is painful
on pressure near its upper part only. Percussion is dull over the tumour; pulse
90; states that for three months past he has not lost in strength. There is slight
oedema. To have two pills of iodide or iron morning and evening.'

• •

This unfortunate man probably had a 'chronic' leukaemia—called so because the course is less rapid than 'acute'. The large 'tumour' was almost certainly an enormous spleen. Normally the spleen cannot be felt for it is tucked up behind the ribcage on the left. Its precise function is unknown, but removal in adult life is rarely associated with problems, although in childhood there is an increased risk of infection with a bacteria known as the pneumococcus.

Some thirteen years earlier Thomas Hodgkin of Guy's Hospital reported six cases of a condition which had appeared to behave like one another, and to look similar at post-mortem. These he believed to be a form of cancer of lymph glands. Some of these cases would not today be called Hodgkin's disease since this is now a well recognized entity, and today most are curable while in Thomas Hodgkin's time, there was no useful treatment.

Throughout history, the knife was the dominant treatment for many an unwanted lesion. Applications, poultices, bleeding, diets, and other unpalatable practices were at different times, although usually ineffective, of variable fashion.

The grand era of the apothecaries began when chemicals were found to have some therapeutic effect, but with the exception of the occasional anecdote, cancers remained unresponsive.

Radiotherapy

The arrival of a new means of treating cancer had to await the beginning of the twentieth century. X-rays were discovered on 8 November, 1895 by Wilhelm Conrad Röntgen in his laboratory at the Physical Institute of the University of Wurtzburg in Germany. He showed that the X-rays could penetrate objects. The impact of this discovery was enormous. It is difficult to conceive today of a hospital which did not have the wide range of diagnostic procedures which are dependent on X-rays. However, the discovery of radioactivity came six months later and was made in Paris on 1 March 1896 by Antoine-Henri Becquerel. Pierre and Marie Curie reported the discovery of radium in 1898. It was these separate discoveries, each remarkable in their own right, which paved the way for modern radiotherapy.

Techniques of treatment evolved in the early decades of this century and these were largely intended to reduce a tumour in size and to control tumour growth. However in 1950 a classic report was presented which suggested the curative potential of radiotherapy in the treatment of Hodgkin's disease. A new modality for cancer treatment was well established.

Chemotherapy

The medieval apothecaries and alchemists were correct in their beliefs that drugs might influence disease, but their expectations were premature. In the early 1900s Paul Ehrlich discovered that an arsenic compound had antisyphilitic activity, earning him the title of the 'saviour of the race'. This did not compare with the discovery of sulpha drugs, which came after observing that a dye, prontosil red, protected mice against certain bacteria. No drugs active against cancer were discovered until the 1940s. The discovery of one of the first, 'mustine' was dramatic and had far-reaching effects. In the winter of 1943 the allies had a somewhat tenuous hold on southern Italy. On the night of 3 December, enemy bombers attacked the harbour of Bari. Only four ships were hit with high explosive bombs, but their cargo of explosives and fuel produced cataclysmic detonations which blew up a further sixteen ships. In the corner of the harbour was a Liberty ship loaded with 100 tons of mustard gas. This suddenly lifted with a gigantic explosion and disappeared. The gas release was not noticed, but over the ensuing days the terrible consequences became apparent. Through the careful observations of one particular doctor, an American, Colonel John Alexander, the effects of the gas were documented in remarkable detail. As a result, it was realized that bone marrow and lymph node tissue were so markedly affected, that perhaps nitrogen mustards could be used to treat cancers of these tissues. Much work was later needed to prove this, but in the event, this was the first discovery of a remarkably useful family of anticancer drugs. Despite the appalling tragedy of the incident in Bari harbour, it was there that success in another war—that against cancer—began.

The importance of the discovery of these and the many drugs which have followed cannot be estimated. Here was the turning point, for at last there was some means, albeit primitive at first, of helping the patient with disseminated cancer. Other drugs related to vitamins were shown to have an effect on leukaemia. And so began an era in which we have seen a revolution in the attitude to the patient with advanced cancer from one of desperate impotence, to one of constructive realism. While the former fuelled despair, the latter has led to undreamed of progress which continues to the benefit of each new patient who is diagnosed.

A quite different class of drugs—the hormones and antihormones which alter the environment in which the cells are bathed—have also been shown to have useful effects in certain cancers. Other related drugs with greater activity are bound to follow.

Immunotherapy

When it was realized that it was possible to immunize against infection, it was inevitable that attempts would be made to immunize against cancer. Using the body's immunity to destroy cancer cells was called 'immunotherapy'. The first attempts happened as early as 1895. As more and more was learned about the immune system, so enthusiasm for immunotherapy rose. All sorts of concoctions were used, antibodies were raised in other animals by injecting them with cancer tissues, direct injections of cancer tissue were given, either alone or with bacteria, which it was hoped would stimulate the immune response. A whole mythology grew up around different methods of immunotherapy—none can really be said to be more than of research interest. However a more scientific approach to immunotherapy has been explored in the last few years. It has used highly specific antibodies to target substances found only in certain tumour cells. This technique requires very sophisticated laboratory methods, and although theoretically very exciting, has failed to live up to expectations.

Only recently has interest focused on ways in which our normal biology may be modified by drugs. The so called 'biological response modifiers' includes substances such as interferons which occur in all of us, but which can now be manufactured in large quantities. Although regarded as new, interferon was first discovered in 1956, but only recently has the technology been available to produce enough pure material to consider its use in clinical practice. It is, however, not the last drug to be discovered, but the first of a completely new generation of drugs, and so not yet part of history.

3 Some cancer statistics

A population explosion, apparently so much a feature of our time, really began in the nineteenth century. Before this, plague, famine, and wars had a controlling effect on population size which was balanced to an increasing degree by organizational changes, and the evolution of new developments in agricultural practice. In the developing world general improvement in sanitation and nutrition made a substantial impact on health so that infant mortality fell, allowing more people to reach reproductive age. In addition, once common causes of death such as tuberculosis had become treatable so reducing morbidity, and eventually were curable. The discovery of antibiotics which made this possible removed the life-threatening implications of common infections. As a consequence, life expectancy has risen from around 40 years in the last century, to exceed 70 years at the present time.

An inevitable outcome of an enlarging, ageing population is the emergence of diseases which increase in frequency with age; degenerative diseases, heart disease, strokes, and cancer have become increasingly important challenges to modern medicine. In Europe and other Western societies, approximately 1 per cent of the population dies each year. Cancer, heart disease and strokes account for nearly three quarters of these deaths, while diseases of the respiratory system, accidents, and congenital disorders, account for most of the remainder. As might be expected, deaths occur more frequently with increasing age, but cancer is only second to accidents as a cause of death in children.

Fifty years ago, one in nine deaths was from cancer. Today the figure is nearer to one in five. This apparent increase is not real, but related primarily to the impact of antibiotics, which have reduced infectious disease from being a major cause of death to one accounting for only about 1 per cent of all deaths.

In the developing world, where there are deficiencies of nutrition, problems of public health, and limited medical resources, deaths from infection and malnutrition are much more common, so that cancer appears significantly less of a problem, accounting for about 1 in 20 deaths. Of course the difference is artificial since the expectation of life is also less, and as resources become more widely available, so we can expect a substantial increase in the relative number of cancer patients.

A few definitions are useful.

Incidence—the number of cases which occur in a given population over its lifespan. As an example, malignant melanoma in the UK population occurs in about one person out of a hundred thousand.

Prevalence—the number of people with cancer at any given time within a geographical area or defined population. People move around the country, some die, others are born, so that the number of cases found in one hundred thousand people within one area will differ substantially from the incidence.

Mortality—is the incidence of death. For any given population this will, over time, be 100%. It is more usefully expressed as the number of deaths in a given year as a total; by cause; or some other characteristic, such as: by diagnosis; by age; by sex; or a combination of these.

Morbidity—describes the consequences of illness in terms of 'unwellness'. Cold may cause mild morbidity while pneumonia may produce severe morbidity or even death.

Epidemiology—is the study of disease distribution in different population groups. The objectives are to identify causes and groups who are at high risk.

In long-term studies, changes in incidence and the mortality may give clues about the causation of disease. However decades may have to pass before some consequences, such as those resulting from the Chernobyl accident, can be identified.

About one in three of us will develop cancer at some time during our lives. Clearly cardiovascular disease and accidents are also a major cause of morbidity (that is 'sickness') but as later chapters make clear, much of the morbidity caused by cancer can be reversed. The impact of modern cancer care on cancer mortality is clear from the difference between the incidence rate of one in three, and the mortality of one in five. This contrasts with heart disease where cure is unusual. The causes of death from cancer in men and women in the UK and USA are shown in table 1.

Those planning the delivery of healthcare need to know the size of a medical problem in their districts in order to allocate resources. They are interested in prevalence rather than incidence, although were the incidence to rise so too would the prevalence, unless effective treatment were rapidly available. In a population of 60 million (about the size of the United Kingdom) there are approximately one million people alive with cancer at any one time. In a district of 300 000 people there are about 1500 new cancer registrations and about 900 deaths from cancer each year. When looked at in terms of hospital referrals, these figures can be very misleading. The reality is that any family doctor may see some cancers very infrequently indeed.

A common question posed is 'How likely am I to get cancer?'. That risk can be crudely calculated but is largely meaningless to any one individual. Another question 'Am I more likely to get cancer than my friend or neighbour?', needs information derived by epidemiologists from the study of risk factors for cancer in different populations. Many different factors are involved to a greater or lesser extent. Examples of a few are: age, sex, occupation, environment, diet, ethnic origin, whether a smoker or non-smoker and for breast cancer whether the mother or sister/s had breast cancer.

A very widely recognized causal factor is tobacco smoking. Snuff taking was recognized as early as the eighteenth century to cause cancer of the nose, and later that century, cancer of the lip was identified to be associated with pipe smoking. During the twentieth century there has been a vast increase in cancer of the lung in the Western world, but it was not until the 1940s that this was established beyond reasonable doubt to be due to the increased use of tobacco products.

Cancer of the larynx, pancreas, kidney, and bladder have also been attributed to cigarette smoking, indeed this has been said to contribute to 35 per cent of all cancer deaths. If this was not enough the risk of a fatal or non-fatal episode due to coronary heart disease is 60–70 per cent greater in male smokers than non-smokers, and about 70 per cent of cases of chronic obstructive airways disease (such as chronic bronchitis) are associated with smoking. In addition maternal smoking during pregnancy is related to an increase in early foetal and neonatal deaths. The risks are now realized to extend to non-smokers who share air space (or smoke space) with smokers (so called 'passive smoking').

Table 1 UK and US cancer deaths by site expressed as a percentage of total cancer deaths

Type of cancer	1992 (UK)		1993 (US) *Estimated deaths	
	Male	Female	Male	Female
Oral (pharynx)	1	0.3	1	0.5
Oesophagus	4	3	3	1
Stomach	7	5	3	2
Colon/Rectal	11	12	10	11
Pancreas	4	4	4	5
Liver	1	1	2	2
Lung	30	16	34	22
Malignant melanoma	1	1	2	1
Breast	–	19	–	18
Cervix uteri	–	2	–	2
Corpus uteri	–	1	–	2
Ovary	–	6	–	5
Prostate	11	–	13	–
Urinary (bladder/kidney)	7	4	5	3
Leukaemia	3	2	4	3
NHL	3	3	4	4
Multiple myeloma	1	1	2	2
Total all sites excluding non-melanoma skin cancer	100	100	100	100

Cancer-causing chemicals have been mentioned earlier. The best known of these is found in cigarette smoke, and there is evidence that some dietary and other environmental factors (such as exposure to certain mineral dusts, chemicals, radiation, and some viruses) may contribute to the incidence of cancer. Epidemiological surveys have occasionally shown an abnormal concentration of cases of a particular cancer, in a geographical locality. This so called 'clustering' is a stimulus to search for a causative factor. The most recent example is the slight increase in leukaemia found in children living near to the Sellafield nuclear processing plant. The question asked is whether radiation might be responsible for the apparent increase in the number of cases of leukaemia. To link this positively with radiation is not possible, but since the major external factor distinguishing this area is the nuclear plant, the link assumption is made. Another theory is that the development of an isolated community may be a factor. However, the difficulties in relating cause and effect can be seen only too clearly in this example.

Radiation has long been known to be associated with an increased risk of cancer. Early workers with X-rays had a higher incidence of skin cancer. Those handling radioactive materials, i.e. extracting radium from pitch blende, or as happened later, painting watch dials with luminous paint containing radium and thorium, developed other cancers including leukaemia and bone cancer.

The most horrific mass exposure to radiation occurred following the explosions of atom bombs at Hiroshima and Nagasaki. Apart from the deaths caused directly by the explosions more deaths than would be predicted have been seen from leukaemias and some solid cancers twenty or more years later.

It is now realized that risks from radiation exposure differ with the type of radiation and with the rate of exposure. Those who received massive doses of radiation from the atomic bombs received the whole dose in one huge burst, or one exposure (called a 'fraction'). Chronic exposure seems to have very different risks, for example when radiation is used in a controlled way for treatment and relatively low doses are given in many exposures (fractions), the risk of causing a second malignancy is known to be almost zero.

Interest in the environmental hazards of radiation has been heightened by the release of radiation from the Chernobyl Nuclear Reactor disaster. Thousands of reindeer were slaughtered in Finland since their carcasses had well above the acceptable levels of radioactivity. Unfortunately prevailing winds carried rain clouds over northern Europe, so that Scotland and north Wales also received a dousing of radioactive material and here too, animals had to be slaughtered and the carcasses disposed of. Some radioactive materials are taken up by the vegetation and so will be recycled to a limited degree which means that exposure is not limited to one season alone. Predictions have been made about the possible small increase in cancer that may eventually result from the accident, but these are unlikely to equal the local casualties caused at the time.

It is known that some rocks used in building, particularly granite, have low emissions of radioactivity. If this causes cancer then 'clustering' of cases of disease increased by radioactivity such as leukaemia, might be expected in those regions where granite is frequently found as a major building material. Cornwall is a prime example, but no such clustering is found. These facts are largely reassuring, but as the consequences of a radiation effect in the long term are not directly measurable, any known radiation exposure will continue to cause sporadic public anxiety.

Clustering of certain cancers has also been reported in other situations: the recognition of cancer of the nasal sinus in wood workers led to a change in industrial practice; cancer of the bladder in the dye industry led to recognition that certain aromatic dyes are carcinogenic. Unsubstantiated reports were made that the incidence of lung cancer appeared higher on the opposite side of gas works from the prevailing wind, and others that Hodgkin's disease seemed to have occurred with a greater than expected frequency in a local population. Chance probably accounts for most of these observations but modern information systems will allow each of these to be examined repeatedly over the course of time.

Another form of clustering is that which occurs not in space (i.e. geographically), but over time. Many years ago, some people with Hodgkin's disease who where not geographically associated, were found to have shared common periods of time in relative association with one another, for example some were at the same schools. The significance of this finding is still debated since no causal factor is known for Hodgkin's disease, but as it may occur in both identical twins, and in more than one member of a family, a complex relationship between inherited and environmental factors has been postulated. Such associations must however be very rare, as family links between people with Hodgkin's disease are infrequent.

Very rarely (so rarely, that whenever they are found interested groups seek to document them in detail), families are found in which there is a very high incidence of cancer. Such cancer families, are very different from the family in which one or two members have cancer. Clear genetic links are now known to exist and study of family members means that those who have a higher than normal risk of developing the cancer can often be identified. This may help to identify those in whom some preventative measures or screening, may be helpful. Genetic counselling can be very helpful to such families especially in identifying the risks to offspring. Since the incidence of cancer in the population as a whole is one in three people, then many families are likely to have one or more member who will develop cancer and this alone does not identify a cancer family. Cancer families are very rare. Some may have associated congenital conditions such as multiple polyps of the colon.

It is inevitable that many wonder whether cancer can be contagious but there is no evidence whatsoever that cancers are infectious—quite the contrary, the overwhelming evidence is that they are not. However infectious hepatitis—hepatitis B—which is rare in Britain, but very common in the Far East, is known to produce liver damage which in some people leads to an increased risk of cancer of the liver—hepatoma. This is one of the commonest cancers in China and the bordering countries.

At the present time, when most cancers are found with increasing age, it is the improving health of the nation and the consequent expansion of the ageing population which inevitably means that cancer will be with us as a significant health problem for the foreseeable future.

4   Screening for cancer

The idea of a universal screening test for cancer may sound very attractive. Before you become too enthusiastic let us examine not only the implications of such a test but the problems which are likely to surround it. Cancers appear at different ages and in different people so that the tests would need to be done at intervals during their lives and this, of course, raises the question as to how often the tests should be performed.

Although we have cheated slightly in talking about a universal test, it is very likely that no such thing will ever be discovered, for cancers arise in different tissues and these have very different characteristics so that screening tests are most likely to have to be individualized for different cancers. This means that any one person would have to have several screening tests performed at intervals if the screening procedure is to be useful. Then we come to the question of how sensitive any one of these tests might be. If the screening test uses X-rays to detect a lump then each has to be a critical size, probably involving hundreds of millions of cells before it is big enough to be seen. Equally, if the test depends on something the tumour produces in the blood there have to be enough cells producing the substance in levels which can be detected. There is one particular tumour of the testicle called a teratoma which produces a substance called alpha-fetoprotein and although this might be a very useful test for screening, a significant number of people with teratoma do not have detectable levels in their blood. Furthermore it is not absolutely specific for teratoma.

After reading this your enthusiasm for a universal cancer test may be beginning to flag and unfortunately there are also several other problems which you should consider. One of these is that in order to screen for cancer you will need to do the tests on many people who are entirely healthy. This has two serious consequences. The first is that people who would not have given a thought to illness or something as serious as cancer are introduced to a worry which they would not otherwise have had. The second factor relates to the question of cost, for most of the expense will be related to testing people whose results will be entirely negative, so that the cost of detecting a cancer is very much higher than the actual cost of the particular test.

These various issues are well recognized and have led to the realization that rather than target the whole population a screening test might be made more valuable if people at higher than average risk of cancer could be identified and the screening test applied to them.

In recent years a huge amount of interest has been generated into whether particular cancers might be screened for. Before doing so, however, it has been recognized that a number of key criteria must be satisfied before introducing the screening process into the health care system. Some of the most important principles are as follows:

1. It is not appropriate to screen for conditions unless there is an effective treatment available to deal with them.

2. The cancer should be a significant problem in the community.

3. There should be a suitable screening test.

4. Groups at higher risk of the cancer should be identifiable to avoid the need for screening the whole population.

5. The optimal interval between tests should be identified.

The easier a screening test is to carry out the more likely are the target populations to comply. At the moment there is no test which a person can carry out in their own home, most unfortunately require a visit to the doctor's surgery or to the hospital which many find intimidating.

The huge interest in screening is fuelled by the thought that if one can identify cancer early enough then treatment is more likely to be effective. A confusing feature which we cannot ignore is that while screening may improve the early detection of all cancers, it may only benefit the treatment of certain sub-groups (so far unidentified) of cancers. What this is saying is that not only do we have to test many healthy people who gain no benefit from the screening test in order to identify those who have cancer, but that we also may have to test many people with cancer in order to identify a specific sub-group of people who are most likely to benefit from early diagnosis. It seems very probable that the latter is true. Although there have been a number of large studies of screening in breast cancer which have demonstrated a clear enough advantage from breast screening for a national breast cancer screening programme to be introduced, the benefits are not dramatically obvious and require very large clinical trials to show the benefit.

An early approach which one might have assumed to be a useful screening measure was the mass miniature chest X-ray screening programme which was set up to detect diseases of the lungs, in particular tuberculosis and lung cancer. However, investment was not thought sufficiently useful and the programme was abandoned.

There are now two cancers for which national screening programmes exist-breast cancer and cancer of the cervix.

Breast cancer

A study in New York was started in 1964 to examine the role of clinical examination and mammography as screening methods for breast cancer. It involved 62 000 women aged 40–64. This Health Insurance Plan (HIP) trial and later Scandinavian studies prompted the setting up of the NHS breast screening programme. In 1992/3 1.6 million women (one third of those aged 50–64) in the UK were invited to participate. Nearly 1.2 million responded and of these about 63 000 were recalled for further investigation which led to finding 6597 cancers.

An expectation of this screening programme is that cancers will be picked up earlier and this was borne out by finding one in five which were one centimetre or less in diameter. A recent large Swedish analysis of five studies of screening in over a quarter of a million women followed for 5–13 years showed the largest reduction of breast cancer mortality (29 per cent) among women aged 50–69.

These are very encouraging results and would appear to justify the colossal resources required for this programme but emphasize the need to search for ways of identifying those at greatest risk. Only if this can be done will large numbers of women who stand to gain nothing from screening be spared an unnecessary examination.

Cancer of the cervix

Screening for cancer of the cervix involves taking a smear from the cervix, staining it with special dyes, and then looking at the cells under the microscope. Obviously the smear must be properly taken and from the right area or the cells will not be representative of those around the cervix. In addition the interpretation of the smears cannot be done without appropriate training.

National screening programmes have been active in Europe and North America for over twenty years and have been shown to be effective in a number of countries, although not by means of strictly controlled trials. The frequency of smears and the target population vary from country to country but accumulating evidence suggests that observed increases of incidence and death from cervical cancer would have been worse had there not been a screening programme.

Although there has probably been a real increase in the incidence of cancer of the cervix in younger women under 35 in which the genital wart virus is implicated, it is older women from poor social backgrounds who are more at risk.

Data from Scandinavian studies suggests that if a woman is screened every five years between the ages of 20 and 64 her risk of developing invasive cancer is reduced by over 80 per cent. Making the screening interval three years improves this figure by 7 per cent but almost doubles the number of smears in her lifetime.

Screening for cancer of the cervix is now well established and future programmes are likely to focus on reaching those at greatest risk and on increasing the reliability of all aspects of the programme so that some of the unfortunate episodes of the past where patients with cancer have been tested but either missed or not followed-up are not repeated.

Ovarian cancer

A screening test would be very desirable for cancer of the ovary, but although some cancers result in increased levels of a measurable substance in the blood (CA-125) this is not reliable enough to use for screening. There is some interest in using sophisticated methods of ultrasound. Unfortunately this is very time consuming, depends very much on the skill of the operator and is not yet reliable enough to introduce into a national screening programme.

Cancer of the colon

At the moment there is no general screening programme for bowel cancer. The only practical way to screen large sections of the population is by faecal occult blood tests—testing the stools for minute amounts of blood which are not visible to the naked eye. There are problems with this test. It requires people to test their stools on a regular basis and may not therefore be acceptable to people who have no symptoms; it yields many false positive results and these cause great anxiety and have to be followed-up by further tests; and it is quite expensive.

Despite these difficulties, faecal occult blood tests offer the possibility of picking up colon cancer at an early stage when it is most curable. Trials are now in progress to see whether this test does in practice save lives by detecting substantially more cancers at an earlier stage than are found at present, and to see whether it is practical and acceptable to the general population.

For people who have a strong family history of colon cancer, it may be worthwhile considering the benefit of regular screening over the age of 35–40, with a regular faecal test for occult blood, and possibly regular colonoscopies (see p.42).

5 *How do cancers cause symptoms?*

Those who received a letter from a cancer society in North America some years ago might have been slightly taken aback by the message on the envelope flap which enquired among other things about a change in bowel habit, unusual bleeding, or change in a mole. Of course, although any one of these may be caused by a cancer, they may also result from other problems which are quite unrelated to cancer. There are in fact no symptoms (sensations of which the patient is aware) or signs (which can also be detected by others) which are absolutely diagnostic, which is why investigation eventually has to include removal of tissue and examination under a microscope (a biopsy) as this is the only secure way of proving that cancer is present.

The tumour

Groups of cells which divide and multiply expand the tissue in which they are growing. They may infiltrate widely causing an ill-defined mass or remain fairly localized causing a well circumscribed lump. Either way they can damage normal structures causing loss of function or obstruction.

Any small lump which enlarges will eventually draw attention to itself. If it is deep in the body it may take some time to do so, while if it is in or near the skin it may be found very easily, for example while washing. An abscess results from infection by bacteria causing a collection of pus to accumulate and may enlarge very rapidly causing surrounding inflammation and pain. Some cancers may behave like this but more usually they grow in a discrete way and are initially quite painless. To begin to appreciate how cancers may produce their symptoms, it is necessary to understand the less attractive characteristics of a cancer. These characteristics depend very much on where the cancer starts, for its behaviour is influenced by the tissue from which it arises, and also the organ in which it begins, and especially on whether it is near some anatomically important structure. One of the cancer's unattractive features is that the cancer cells do not grow alongside one another in the regimented and controlled way that normal cells do, so that their blood supply also develops in a rather haphazard way. This means that some parts of the tumour do not receive adequate oxygen and nutrition and may actually die—such 'necrosis' as it is called is a characteristic of some cancers and may actually lead to quite rapid changes in their size. When they are near to a surface, i.e. in the skin or in the intestinal tract (bowel) the dead tissue may slough away resulting in ulcers which can become infected and bleed. In deep tissues a sterile 'abscess' may form which very occasionally may partially heal giving the temporary impression that the tumour is actually getting smaller.

Swelling

This is the most obvious feature of a cancer. Only in leukaemias is swelling not a classical feature, and even then deposition of leukaemic cells in glands, skin, or other tissues may cause swelling.

Different cancers vary enormously in the rate at which they grow. Some may literally take years to grow, while others may appear within a few days. If the swelling develops within a structure such as a breast or in the abdomen and is very slow growing indeed, it may take years to come to notice. Pain is rarely a feature of a small swelling, so often it comes to be found by accident or because it causes some local problem which leads to symptoms in the organ or tissue concerned. Fast growing cancers may ulcerate or cause pain before the developing swelling attracts much attention. The swelling is caused by cancer cells multiplying. Each cell is capable of dividing into two daughter cells. A few calculations show that if each cell divides regularly and no cells break away and die, it will not take very long to achieve the 1000 million cells needed to make a lump the size of the end of the little finger. In practice things are much more haphazard. Normal cells would die very quickly under these conditions, but cancer cells survive rather better and while some certainly do not survive, others do, dividing to produce further cells which accumulate to produce the swelling.

Obstruction

This may involve bowel, airways, blood vessels, and other drainage channels. If a tumour grows to produce a swelling in the wall of a bowel or in a structure like the prostate, blockage to the passage may occur. In the bowel waves of muscular contraction in the wall (peristalsis) push the food along but when this meets a mass in the wall of the bowel the peristalsis becomes more active in an attempt to move the lump along. Some spasm of the bowel wall muscle may lead to stomach pains which do not go away, and to irregularity of bowel motions ranging from diarrhoea to constipation. When obstruction occurs in the upper bowel food may pass with difficulty and so cause nausea, loss of appetite and occasional vomiting. Compression of the urethra (the connecting tube between the bladder and the penis) by a prostatic cancer may make emptying the bladder rather hard work—so much so that it is not emptied properly and leads to a desire to pass urine frequently during the day and night. Of course, enlargement of the prostate without a cancer occurs very commonly with increasing age, and more often than not these symptoms result from a harmless cause which can easily be corrected by surgery. Similarly compression of the tube draining the kidney (the ureter) may eventually lead to the kidney failing on that side.

If a tumour occurs in the lungs and is located in or near the main airway, this can cause shortness of breath or irritation leading to a persistent non-productive cough. Ulceration of the air passages may cause some blood to appear in the phlegm produced on coughing.

Obstruction of a blood vessel may cause no problem at all since there are many channels supplying blood to tissues (arteries) and collecting it from them (veins). Just occasionally a main blood vessel can be involved in which case cramp-like pains are caused in the area supplied by the artery which is obstructed. When a major vein is obstructed other veins under the skin may visibly get larger as they take over the drainage of the area, however when a main vein from a leg is involved tissue fluids may be only incompletely drained and as a consequence the leg may swell. This is a common feature of a 'deep vein thrombosis' which can occur spontaneously, after injury or occasionally after operations, and may be totally unrelated to cancer.

Another feature of cancers is that the newly produced cancer cells do not respect any of the boundaries around them. This means that they may invade blood vessels or nerves which lie close by. Often this may cause little or no problem although infiltration of the cancer cells around certain nerve endings may cause pain. When a large nerve is affected there may be weakness or numbness depending on whether the nerve's function is to send messages to muscle or to receive messages relating to sensation. When these main nerves are damaged by growing cancer there may be both loss of sensation and muscle weakness. This sounds very alarming and often is, even when it is caused by something quite unrelated to cancer, such as disc trouble in the back. The spinal cord contains bundles of nerves grouped together rather like telephone lines and power cables side by side. It can be imagined that damage to these can produce substantial effects.

Should some cancer cells lodge within the brain (this is commoner in the very late stage of cancers than at the beginning) then the problems they cause depend on the site where they are lodged and by how much the lump expands. The effect may range from no apparent damage to that of a serious stroke.

Pain

Everyone is familiar with pain. It is relatively easy to produce and is nature's extremely effective way of drawing attention to an area where all is not well. Sitting in a badly designed chair may produce pain, but usually this disappears quickly when the position is changed. It is the persistence of pain which draws attention to a possible underlying problem. A dental abscess may be excruciatingly painful but relief is almost immediate when the abscess is drained. The pain is caused by pressure from the increased accumulation of infected material. Cancer by causing a swelling may cause pain in this way. Very occasionally in leukaemia the active leukaemia in the bone marrow may cause pain in long bones as the cells continue to multiply in a cavity of limited volume, while in other conditions like myeloma, weakness of a bone at the site of the tumour may result in pain when any pressure is exerted upon it. The body has a very complex and very sophisticated system of nerve endings which register pain so that this sensation may be felt almost anywhere. In addition to pain from the direct pressure of an enlarging tumour, pain may also result indirectly from pressure on other structures lying nearby, or as a result of pressure on or irritation of nerves. Direct irritation of nerve endings is a feature of ulceration.

Change in character

Although this concept is well recognized by clinicians and pathologists it is only commonly known about as something which may occur in moles. This is a very rare event (since most people have a good number of moles and cancer in moles—melanoma—is rare) but when it does occur is seen as a change in the size or appearance of the mole heralding malignant change. This is dealt with on p.168–169.

Alteration in function

The body is a unique world of its own where breakdown of function occurs only rarely. It depends on the symbiosis not only with its own structures, but with the world around it. The bowel contains, for example, about one kilogram of living bacteria which play an essential role in digestion. If the balance is disturbed as may happen when antibiotics are taken, then diarrhoea results because different bacteria take over. Many other factors may alter bowel function and cancer is one of them. A cancer in the wall of a bowel can, as has been described, if low down cause alteration of bowel habit or if high up nausea, vomiting, and loss of appetite. Conditions other than cancer such as inflammation of the bowel or a peptic ulcer may produce exactly similar symptoms. The liver is the body's food factory and is responsible for converting the food we eat into substances the body needs. Without it the body's tissues become starved of energy so that weakness and weight loss occur. Although it is vital for life it is a huge organ and a great deal has to be damaged by cancer tissues before it fails. Similarly as there are two kidneys it is unusual for kidney failure to be a problem but if they both become damaged then the body begins to have difficulty handling the disposal of waste products and excess fluid. Another example where function is altered is in leukaemia. Here the bone marrow (where the blood components are made) works less efficiently because the primitive blood cells do not mature fully and compete with the normal development. As a consequence, three populations of cells which start life in the bone marrow may be reduced in the blood, the red cells which may cause anaemia, the white cells which may lead to an increased risk of infection, and the platelets which may result in an increased risk of bleeding.

Many other bodily functions may be altered by diseases other than cancer but may mimic it— for example, periods may become irregular when fibroids are present or because of hormonal imbalance. When a cancer of the cervix is present irregular bleeding may happen but other symptoms such as pain or discharge may also develop. Certain cancers can actually cause an over-production of normal substances, for example increased mucus in cancers of the bowel. In rather rare cancers a whole range of hormones may be produced in excess and result in symptoms which are thought to be rather bizarre until it is realized that a tumour is present.

Loss of function

This has been discussed in part in relation to alteration in function. Injuries to nerves from whatever cause may result in some loss of function in the organ tissue or limb which they supply. A very important situation is where damage is beginning to occur to the spinal cord. This may result from fracture of a vertebra, poor blood supply to the cord, pressure from a disc, from tumour or injury. Gradual onset of weakness in the legs with or without loss of sensation, plus some difficulty in controlling the bladder and perhaps bowel sphincters, are urgent indications for immediate investigation within 24 hours. Other types of nerve damage may result from all kinds of causes, of which cancer is one. If new problems develop in someone with cancer these will often be attributed to the cancer. Whatever the background this is a problem which needs to be explained and so further investigation is indicated.

Persistence of symptoms

Symptoms which continue over a period of time, especially when they are progressively worsening, are usually an indication that investigation is needed. Cancer may well have nothing to do with such symptoms but as the possibility that cancer may be present is frequently a hidden anxiety it is important to exclude it as a cause. Persistent cough in a heavy smoker may not indicate a cancer, but clearly if other symptoms are present such as increasing shortness of breath, and perhaps blood in the sputum, then investigation is warranted. It is the continuation of symptoms which is the body's way of saying 'here, come and sort this out'. It is *not* a message which says that cancer is present. Indeed, it is the persistence of symptoms from whatever cause which classically persuades someone to visit his or her family doctor.

Bleeding

A bleeding nose is common and only rarely is an indication of anything serious. There is a sensitive patch inside the nose which is full of small fragile blood vessels and will bleed if damaged. In patients who have a tendency to bleed, as may happen in leukaemia, frequent nose bleeds may also occur. Bleeding from other sites when unexpected should be investigated, but it should be remembered that cancer is just one of many possible causes. There are many reasons why ulceration of the bowel may occur, but whatever the cause this can lead to blood loss which, if fresh, is noted when the bowel is emptied. If bleeding occurs from an ulcer high in the bowel the blood may be partially digested and so appear black—the so called 'malaena' stool. Bleeding into the motions may result from haemorrhoids or inflammation of the bowel. Similarly, an ulcer of the urinary tract may cause blood in the urine. Bleeding into the urine may result from cystitis—a bladder infection. Coughing up blood as sometimes happens in lung cancer may actually follow a bleeding nose resulting in blood draining down the back of the throat.

Menstruation is entirely normal, but obviously bleeding after the menopause needs to be investigated.

Symptoms such as those described here can be very worrying and obviously need investigation. Unfortunately it is not possible to be reassured until the cause is known, which is a very good reason for going to see the doctor promptly.

6 *Tests for cancer and how cancer is investigated*

•••

General principles

The most important part of any investigation where cancer is suspected is first to prove the diagnosis. To do this, it is essential to take a sample (a biopsy) of the suspect tissue, and then a pathologist will examine it under the microscope (histological examination). Sometimes it is possible to take such a 'biopsy' under local anaesthetic, as for example when a piece of skin is to be removed or a sample of bone marrow. Often the biopsy is taken during an operation when tissue is removed from what appears to be an abnormal area. Usually the abnormal area would be removed in entirety, but when this is not possible because the tumour is too extensive or involves vital structures, a representative piece of tissue is biopsied for the pathologist to examine. Glands under the arm and in the neck, and where the tissue to be removed is bulky, are often most easily removed when the patient has a general anaesthetic, in which case an overnight stay in hospital may be necessary.

Biopsy of the liver and kidneys has long been possible under local anaesthetic using specially designed needles. Modern techniques of ultrasound or using a body scanner allow an operator to take samples with remarkable precision from deep in the body without the need for a general anaesthetic. The biopsy taken with these needles is very useful when 'positive', but the amount of tissue is much smaller than would be taken by the surgeon so that if a sample is reported as 'normal', it may in the end be necessary to ask for an open biopsy to be sure that an abnormality has not been missed. By freezing biopsy tissue immediately it has been removed it is possible to look at the material very quickly (in under an hour), and when cancer is obvious, this can be most helpful. This technique is used quite frequently to decide on the extent of an operation needed. However the best preservation of material requires careful preparation so that a full report cannot usually be issued in less than two to three days. Once a cancer has been diagnosed conclusively, the pathologist may want to examine the specimen further using special stains. This involves using different chemical dyes or labelled antibodies which recognize certain substances found only, or more commonly, in cells of a particular kind. The need for this further examination comes from the fact that it is now possible to identify sub-types of particular cancers. Some sub-types behave differently—for example lung cancer can be sub-divided into at least five main varieties by the pathologist—and if as sometimes occurs, there is uncertainty about whether the cancer started in the lung or is a metastasis from a cancer arising in a completely different tissue, special stains may be very helpful in deciding this question and in making the final diagnosis. In the case of bone marrow biopsies, the bone calcium has to be removed before sections of the marrow can be cut, stained, and examined. All this means that there may be delays of up to a week before the results of a bone marrow biopsy can be known.

Sometimes it is possible to dislodge enough cells from a suspected cancer by scraping or washing, so that a diagnosis can be made after these have been stained and examined under the microscope. A cervical smear is prepared in this way, as are washings from the bronchus (the tubes to the lungs) taken at 'bronchoscopy' (see p.41). Similarly, fluid from a cyst or body cavity can be examined for 'malignant cells'. Examples of these are breast cysts and fluid from the lung cavities (pleural effusion) or fluid in the abdominal cavity (ascites), both of which may accumulate as a consequence of illness.

A record of how the illness became apparent including associated medical events, those occurring throughout life and any pertinent facts, form an essential part of the medical 'history', which is recorded for every patient. As most people have eventful lives in one way or another the doctor's skill is, with the help of the patient, to elicit the important facts. By the time a diagnosis is made, most patients will probably have had several full *clinical examinations*. The doctor will carry out a general examination similar to that for insurance purposes, but in addition he will be looking for any evidence of cancer, such as abnormal lumps or bumps, or of the consequences of a cancer. Since cancers may cause literally any clinical consequence, including such widely differing features as enlarged glands draining the area of the cancer, distension of the bowel, enlargement of the liver or spleen, alteration in the way the veins drain, swelling of a limb or of the face and neck, even abnormalities of heart valves and changes in vision, clearly the examination has to be careful and thorough. This preliminary assessment helps the doctor to decide what path of investigation he should follow.

Certain investigations are fairly routine as part of the initial assessment. An early blood sample which is collected from the vein in the arm may be used for the following tests.

Full blood count—the blood contains three main types of cells or parts of cells. Firstly there are red cells which contain haemoglobin, the red pigment which carries oxygen. Shortage of red cells results in anaemia. Secondly there are white cells—several different types of white cells are found but the most important are the granulocytes which fight infection by bacteria, and lymphocytes which are concerned primarily with immunity. Thirdly there are platelets—these are cell fragments which plug gaps in blood vessels to prevent bruising or haemorrhage.

Urea and electrolytes—Sodium, potassium, and urea are usually measured. Since blood is our own internal medium and we have evolved from creatures which lived in the sea, salt solution, in particular the levels of sodium and potassium salts, are fairly critical within the blood. Sickness of body cells will effect these levels as will a failure of kidney function, since they and urea (one of the body's waste products) are excreted via the kidneys.

Liver function tests—the liver is the body's factory which converts the constituents of foodstuff to produce materials essential for many functions. It is also a major energy source. Eight to ten substances are measured routinely, and these can give a good indication of whether the liver is functioning normally. Often these tests include the calcium level which is influenced by levels of protein in the blood and may be raised in certain uncommon circumstances even when the bones are not obviously compromised.

Many special blood tests exist which may only be used when certain rare cancers are suspected, for example alpha-fetoprotein (which is also raised in normal pregnancy), and beta-HCG, both of which are raised in rare tumours of germ cell tissue i.e. the reproductive tissue of the testes and ovaries. Another compound, 5HIAA, is raised in carcinoid tumours (see p.134).

X-rays

Having an X-ray is now a very straightforward process which generally means standing in front of, or lying down, over a plate which contains X-ray film. The actual exposure lasts for less than a second and delivers only a minuscule dose of radiation. A plain chest X-ray is a most useful examination. On it can be seen the size and outline of the heart, the great vessels, the trachea, the oesophagus, bony structures including ribs, clavicles, and scapuli (the vertebrae are often obscured by the central structures namely the heart, great vessels, trachea, and oesophagus), and the lung tissues. Enlarged glands in the middle of the chest (the mediastinum) or at the root of the lungs cannot be detected by clinical examination, but can readily be detected on chest X-ray.

It is, of course, possible to X-ray any part of the body. X-rays of bones may reveal fractures, tumours, or secondary tumours (metastases) in bone, or indeed other structural abnormalities; however, such X-rays tell us nothing about the function of the bone marrow where blood is produced.

X-rays of soft tissues—the best known of these is the mammogram (see p.92–93).

X-rays of the abdomen—these are taken in the same fashion as a chest X-ray, although they are also commonly taken with the patient lying down. The X-ray only shows the bowel where it is full of gas, but it does show the bones of the back and pelvis, and the outline of the liver, kidneys, and spleen. Various changes can be seen such as occurs when the bowel is immobilized and so not pushing the food along, and may be very helpful in making a diagnosis. For a more detailed examination of intracavitary structures it is necessary to have a contrast X-ray. This may require a period of fasting (often over-night) and require contrast material to be swallowed in order to show the oesophagus, stomach, duodenum, and small bowel (barium swallow, barium meal, and follow through). A glass full of bland material is swallowed after a cupful of crystals which helps to distribute the barium in the stomach. Then, using a special couch, the radiologist moves the patient and views the bowel using a television linked X-ray, as the contrast moves down the gut. He can then take permanent X-ray pictures at various points to record the image at a critical point.

Barium enema—the large bowel has to be empty for this examination. The preparation takes about two days and involves modifying the diet, avoiding iron tablets, bran, or proprietary laxatives and then taking special laxatives provided by the X-ray department. In order to coat the bowel with barium a small nozzle is inserted into the back passage, barium and air are passed in and the first X-rays taken. The patient is moved to a different position to encourage the contrast to coat the rectum and then the whole of the large bowel which lies rather like a drooped necklace hung from the corners of the top of the abdomen. This very useful X-ray can show the outline of the bowel and whether it is dilated or narrowed but also it may show up abnormalities in the bowel movements.

Cholecystogram—a radio-opaque dye is injected into a vein. This is concentrated through the liver and then drains from this via the bile duct to be collected in the gall bladder. A straightforward X-ray of the abdomen will then show up the gall bladder. The most common finding of all is stones. Cancers of the bile duct and gall bladder are very rare indeed.

Contrast medium can be injected into veins—a *venogram*—and arteries—an *arteriogram*—to show blocks in the vessels. It is possible, by entering an artery in the groin, to feed a catheter back up the main artery to enter small arteries virtually anywhere, and so to show the blood supply of a tumour. This has been considered a possibly useful way of delivering drug treatment, but the results have not justified the introduction of this technique into current practice.

A technique useful for showing changes in lymph glands which may not be apparent on bodyscanner examination is the *lymphangiogram*. It is now less commonly used but can be valuable for looking at the lymph glands at the back of the abdomen. In order to do this a small amount of green dye is injected between the toes. This helps to locate the lymphatic channels on the back of the feet. These channels run up below the skin of the legs via the lymph glands in the groin, and then to lymph glands alongside the main blood vessels in the abdomen. Finally, the lymph draining from the abdomen leaves via a larger vessel called the 'thoracic duct', which drains into the main blood vessel leading to the heart. Once the lymphatics on the foot have been identified, contrast can be injected. This contrast then slowly tracks up the lymphatics to the glands in the abdomen. Once this has entered the glands they can be seen on a standard X-ray of the abdomen, and as the dye stays for some months, repeated X-rays are possible so that changes in the abdominal glands can be seen easily. As with other X-rays of the abdomen this X-ray requires bowel preparation beforehand. The hospital will give instructions on taking laxatives followed by a period of starvation so that the overlying bowel does not seriously interfere with the pictures. This is a lengthy technique for it often takes an hour or so before the contrast is running into each leg, and as lymph fluid moves much less rapidly than blood in arteries and veins, it is necessary to come back a day later for X-rays to be taken of the glands in the abdomen.

An *intravenous urogram, IVU,* (also known as an *intravenous pyelogram, IVP*) is used to look at the kidneys and also the tubes that drain from these to the bladder (the ureters). In order to do this a push injection of contrast dye is given into a vein and as this is excreted through the kidneys it is possible to see the whole drainage system on X-ray examination. Very occasionally, a large mass in the abdomen may obstruct the ureters or push them to one side—in this case an IVP may be very useful. In addition the kidneys are well outlined during this technique, so the kidney itself may be examined closely. It is not uncommon to feel a flush when contrast is given into a vein. Apart from annoyance at the length of the procedure, the main complaint after lymphangiography is of taking on a distinct green hue. This makes one look rather like an announcer on a badly adjusted television set, but rapidly passes. It may however be disconcerting for relatives who fear that the patient is iller than they first realized.

Another useful way of learning about organs within the abdomen non-invasively, is by using *ultrasound*. This technique requires particular skill from the operator but can be most helpful. It is possible to look at the different organs and to identify even quite small lumps. It is now so precise, that needle biopsy can be carried out, under ultrasound guidance, of lumps deep within the abdomen. Ultrasound examination of breast lumps and of the testes has become routine and may help to avoid the need for more invasive investigation.

The most sophisticated use of diagnostic X-ray comes in *CT (computed tomography) scanning*. Here the patient is slowly moved through a ring-shaped device which has X-ray tubes at one side and a number of sensors on the other. By measuring the X-ray emission at different points around the ring (and these vary as a result of the different densities of the tissues through which the X-rays have passed), and then using a powerful computer to relate the readings to one another, a picture can be built up of that part of the body which

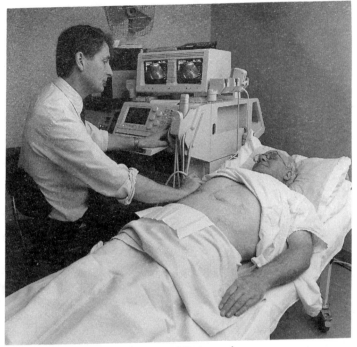

Figure 1 Ultrasound.

lies within the ring. In effect these slices show the structures very much as they would look if the body were sliced through at that point. It is very valuable to be able to repeat these sections as little as one or even half a centimetre apart. Any distortion of tissues can be seen and the precise location of a tumour may very easily be visualized. In order to obtain a slice with fine detail the body must be still, and as for a chest X-ray, breathing should stop while the pictures are generated. Older machines required people to do so for as long as 20–24 seconds which was difficult for the very young, the elderly, or profoundly ill. Now only 3–4 seconds are required, making the examination a great deal easier.

This machinery is not particularly useful for making a diagnosis of cancer—often that is relatively straightforward—but it can be most helpful in watching and monitoring the effect of treatment. Once the

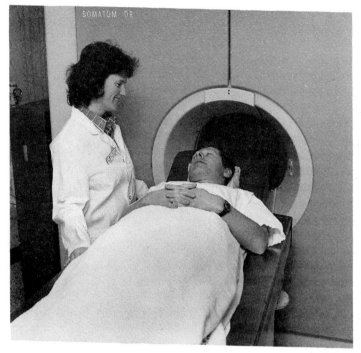

Figure 2 CT scan.

location of the tumour is known it is not necessary to have a scan of the whole body, and few sections or 'cuts' at the level specified can be done very quickly and give all the information that is necessary.

Magnetic resonance imaging (*MRI*) used to be called nuclear magnetic resonance (NMR), and instead of X-rays uses powerful magnetic forces. Special sensors measure the recovery time of the effects of the magnetic forces on tissues. A rather different picture is built up than comes from the CT body scanner, and although it is extremely useful for neurological examinations as yet its value in cancer management is less well established. One of the problems is that tumours arising from a particular tissue do not necessarily show a greater difference from the original tissue, for example tumour deposits in the spleen may show up well on CT scanning but not be visible on MRI. Even when the magnet is switched off there is still an immensely powerful magnetic force so that all iron containing metal objects must be removed before entering the MRI room. This also applies to credit cards which can be wiped clean!

Nuclear medicine is so called because it uses radioactive isotopes to localize abnormalities. Different isotopes are used in different ways in order to show up the tissue which is to be examined. Usually the isotope is given by injection into a vein, time is allowed for it to be taken up in the organ or tissue in question, and then the area (or the whole body if necessary) is moved under a special 'camera' which measures the emitted radiation and records an anatomical plot of the area showing where the radiation is high or low. This way 'cold' or 'hot' spots can be identified. The pattern of change requires an expert interpretation, for example, simple bruising of bone can produce a hot spot which can be very misleading if one is looking for secondaries in bone. As more and more is understood about the special metabolic behaviour of some tumours, so this can be turned to advantage when it comes to scanning with isotopes. A rare tumour of children—neuroblastoma, and an even rarer tumour of adults—phaeochromocytoma, both take up a compound called MIBG (meta-iodobenzylguanidine). This can be tagged with an isotope and the extent of the tumour and indeed its location can be recorded. In certain very special circumstances a much higher dose of radiation can be given to kill the cells which take up the compound, but so far this is experimental.

Endoscopy

Fibre-optics have transformed the way in which doctors can look into cavities. A system of lenses linked to bundles of glass fibres allow vision through a flexible tube to a point which may be three feet or more away. In the past, corners limited the distance which could be examined.

Bronchoscopy is the examination of the passages to the lungs. Using a rigid examination tube the examination was confined to the main airway and a few of the lower passages. Now with flexible bronchoscopes it is possible to examine far out into the lung itself and to take specimens without difficulty. It is helpful to have the co-operation of the patient, so a mild but very effective sedative is given plus a local anaesthetic to the upper air-passages. The tube can then be passed through the nose. Often the patient is sufficiently alert but also sedated in such a way that they may take an interest in the proceedings.

Oesophagoscopy, gastroscopy, and duodenoscopy describe the examination of the upper bowel, namely the oesophagus (the tube to the stomach), stomach, and duodenum (the tube leading from the stomach and on to the small bowel). A rather large bore instrument is used for this and so more sedation is often given, but many people are awake and ready for a cup of tea within an hour of examination. However, as in all cases where sedatives are used in sufficient doses for memory to be impaired, driving is out of the question until the following day.

Examination of the rectum is part of the routine examinations. Although slightly uncomfortable for the patient, the doctor wearing a lubricated rubber glove, can feel various tissues in the pelvis and satisfy himself from gross examination that all is well.

Sigmoidoscopy involves the examination of the rectum and bowel above it using a rigid tube. This is often possible as an out-patient.

Colonoscopy uses fibre-optic apparatus to examine the whole of the large bowel including the rectum. In order to have the bowel empty, there obviously has to be a period of bowel preparation which involves diet modification and aperients.

Cystoscopy In order to examine the bladder an examination tube is passed up the urethra and then into the bladder where biopsies can also be taken. This examination is usually performed under a light general anaesthetic.

7 *Treatments for cancer*

When treatments for cancers are talked about it is of surgery, radio-therapy, or chemotherapy that most people first think. These are discussed in the following chapter but other treatments such as with hormones or biological agents are mentioned in relation to the treatment of specific cancers.

Surgery

No one can deny the appeal of getting rid of a lump from the body when it should not be there. If an ulcer does not heal or a lump goes on growing their continued presence begins to be seen firstly as something vaguely disturbing, or even offensive, and ultimately as a threat. Surgery in its simplest form, using a knife or cutting implement to remove an unwanted imperfection, has been practised not just for hundreds but for thousands of years. It had to await the discovery of anaesthetics and antiseptics to become the powerful treatment tool that we know today.

Towards the end of the last century the ability to remove even quite large tumours began to have a profound influence on the way surgeons thought about the management of cancers. Great interest was focused on breast cancer, for one reason in particular: that the breast is an appendage and therefore easy to remove. The idea was formulated that this cancer spread in an organized way, first starting in the breast and then spreading into the local lymph glands before disseminating around the body. This dictated that if on examination the tumour appeared not to have spread, the best way to achieve cure was to make the surgery as radical as possible. This meant taking away not only the breast but the muscles of the chest wall underlying it and removing all the lymph glands from the armpit. If this sounds a profoundly mutilating procedure, it was, but had the appeal of being likely to remove all local evidence of cancer. It was an approach used to treat breast cancer all over the world for over half a century.

Some sixty years ago doubt was already voiced about the impact this operation had on survival and subsequent analyses have shown that its main value was in reducing local recurrence and confirmed that it had little or no effect on survival. It is easy, in retrospect, to be critical of these pioneering surgeons but at the time, when neither radiotherapy nor medical treatments were available, theirs was the only treatment with any prospect of success. Had the modern practice of evaluating treatments by clinical trials been available the limitations of radical surgery would have been recognized much earlier, but even if they had been at that time there was very little to offer in its place.

Today surgery is a much more rational science. You will find it mentioned in different parts of this book, playing different roles, each with its own important place in cancer management. As with all aspects of medicine, no procedure is set in stone. Some new approaches, though full of promise, do not stand scrutiny, others become established for many years only to be superseded as new developments take place. Surgery remains the mainstay for the diagnosis and initial treatment of many solid cancers. It has a role in defining the extent of some cancers (staging), in refashioning the body to minimize the effects of a cancer (reconstruction), and in relieving the effects of some cancers (palliation).

Diagnosis

The diagnosis of a cancer needs to be made by looking at a piece of the suspect area for examination under the microscope by a pathologist. Although in some circumstances a smear of cells from the specimen (i.e. blood in the case of leukaemia, fluid from a body cavity, or brushings from an accessible surface of a cancer) may produce enough evidence to make a diagnosis, in most cases it is necessary to remove a piece of tissue. This may require a special operation—a 'biopsy', or tissue may be examined from a whole tumour removed at operation. Nowadays it may be possible to remove enough tissue to make a diagnosis from places quite deep in the body. This can be done under local anaesthetic using ultrasound or X-ray guidance to locate the spot with great accuracy.

Treatment

Where possible, surgery is used to remove a solid cancer as completely as possible. Before doing this the surgeon will probably wish to do a number of tests to ensure that the cancer has not spread to any distant sites, for when this happens surgery may not necessarily be the best treatment. If the cancer appears localized the intention of the surgery will be to remove the visible cancer and any local tissues which might harbour cancer cells. It is not until the tumour is exposed that the surgeon can see just how feasible that will be. Although the very nature of cancers means that it is unlikely that all the cancer will be removed by surgery, the amount of cancer is very substantially decreased and the problems which might have been caused by the cancer are reduced. If the cancer is well localized and slow growing it may never reappear and this is, of course, a major aim of surgery.

Staging

This is the system of defining the disease extent and is different for each cancer. The surgeon's findings at operation are recorded and together with the results of other investigations and those of the pathologist are used to define the extent of the cancer. The scale ranges from very localized to widespread and is helpful both in planning treatment and in giving some indication of outlook. It is no longer usual to do an operation just for staging, but until about ten years ago opening the abdomen was routine in the management of many people with Hodgkin's disease.

Reconstruction

Modern surgery is quite staggering in what can be achieved and these techniques can be very helpful to a cancer patient either in restoring a particular structure (i.e. conserving a limb, rebuilding part of a face, or creating a new bladder) or restoring appearance (i.e. in reconstructing the breast after a mastectomy). The extent to which reconstruction can be carried out or is advisable may depend on the other treatments which are needed and this needs careful thought and good advice.

Palliation

The removal of a lump in someone with widespread cancer which as it grows causes discomfort or other complications is a good reason to consider surgery. Radiotherapy or chemotherapy may also be useful and each situation has to be considered separately. Surgery can be most helpful in a number of situations when the cancer cannot be completely removed. A very good example is when the bowel does not work well because it is bunched up by an area of cancer which is too big or too diffuse to remove. In this case the surgeon can join the ends of the bowel which are unaffected and so allow food to bypass the affected area. If this isn't possible he can bring the end of the unaffected bowel out through the wall of the abdomen and form a 'colostomy'. This is also done for people who have a cancer very low down in the bowel where although the cancer can be removed there is not enough normal bowel remaining above the anus to join the upper piece of bowel to it.

Surgery has a great deal to offer in the management of many cancers and knowing how it is to be used can be very helpful in understanding the overall strategy for dealing with a particular cancer.

Radiotherapy

What is radiotherapy?

Radiotherapy is the use of high-energy rays to kill cancer cells. It is a common treatment for cancer, either on its own or, often, in conjunction with surgery or chemotherapy. Many cancers are sensitive to radiation, and it can be used curatively in many patients. It also has a very valuable part to play in alleviating symptoms.

Everyone is exposed to naturally occurring radiation throughout their lives, from the atmosphere, soil, buildings and food. The levels of background radiation vary from one place to another and generally are not thought to be dangerous. However, in some parts of the world (for example, Pennsylvania, New Jersey, and parts of New York in the United States; the West Country and the Peak District in the UK) the particular geological formation of those areas causes a natural, radioactive gas called radon to seep up from the soil and it may accumulate in the foundations of buildings if they are not properly ventilated. It is now believed that high concentrations of this gas may pose a risk of lung cancer.

Radiation is used for both diagnosis and treatment. X-rays are used to 'photograph' the inside of the body by passing rays through the body onto a sensitive film. Different tissues show up differently on the film, and the picture obtained enables the doctor to check whether anything is awry. The dosage of radiation given with an X-ray is very small and causes no damage to the tissue that it passes through. Nevertheless, the cumulative effect of numerous X-rays could be damaging, and doctors try to limit the number of X-rays needed to make a diagnosis. For treatment purposes, much higher concentrations of high energy radiation are used with the purpose of destroying cells—in this case, cancer cells.

Modern techniques of giving radiotherapy aim to give the maximum possible dose to the tumour while affecting the surrounding tissues as little as possible. However, it may not always be possible to avoid all normal unaffected tissue and there may be some damage to that tissue, which usually recovers after the treatment course is finished. For external radiotherapy, the total dose of radiation needed is broken down into a number of relatively small daily doses (sometimes called fractions). The reason for this is that cancer cells are relatively less able to repair themselves than normal cells; so normal cells have a chance to recover at least part of any damage from radiotherapy between treatments, while the tumour cells become cumulatively weaker.

Radiotherapy is usually given by focusing a beam or a combination of beams of rays at the body from the outside (external beam radiotherapy). This treatment does not make the treated person radioactive, and can be used to treat people, including children, without any risk to them. Another method is to place a source of radiation inside the body for a short period (internal radiotherapy, or brachytherapy). The radioactive source (usually a natural substance which gives off radiation, such as caesium or iridium) can be placed next to or even inside the tumour, giving a very precise dose exactly where it is needed. This method is often used to treat cervical and breast cancers, among others. While the source is in the body, the person is mildly radioactive, but the radioactivity goes as soon as the source is removed. During treatment, certain precautions are taken to ensure that visitors are not exposed to any risk.

One further method of treatment is the use of a drink or injection of a radioactive chemical. It is used when it is known that the part of the body where the cancer lies takes up that particular chemical very readily. The classic case is the treatment of thyroid disease with radioactive iodine. For a few days after the radioactive substance has been given the person is mildly radioactive while it wears off and is excreted from the body.

Why is radiotherapy given?

Radiotherapy is a local treatment—that is, it affects only the part of the body that it is directed at. It is therefore only useful when the cancer is confined to one or only a few sites; if the cancer is very widespread, treatment by radiotherapy is not practical.

Curative treatment

In some cases radiotherapy can be given with a realistic hope of curing the cancer, i.e. with curative intent. There is a maximum limit to the amount of radiotherapy any individual tissue of the body can tolerate, and one of the crucial considerations for radiotherapists is how to avoid exceeding this limit. There are a number of other considerations which also determine whether the treatment is feasible:

- If the primary tumour is very sensitive to radiotherapy. This means that even if the tumour is fairly large, quite a low dose of radiation can be given. The classic case of this is with lymphomas which can be very successfully treated.

- If the tumour is quite sensitive to radiation, and can be destroyed with a lower dose than would cause damage to the normal tissue around it. Skin cancers, for example, can often be successfully treated with radiotherapy because an adequate dose to kill the cancer cells does very little damage to normal tissues. Tumours in the liver, on the other hand, are not very sensitive while the liver itself is very easily damaged by radiation. As a result treatment to destroy liver tumours may cause more damage to the normal liver than is worthwhile in terms of treatment of the cancer.

- Where the tumour lies, and what other organs or structures are nearby. For example a tumour next to the spinal cord is more difficult to treat as the spinal cord needs to be protected from receiving the full dose of radiation, without compromising treatment to the tumour.

- How large the tumour is. It is much easier to give a high dose to a small area than to a large one.

- If the primary tumour has been removed by surgery, but the doctors know that tiny specks of cancer cells have been left behind, radiotherapy after surgery can destroy any microscopic disease.

- If there is cancer in other parts of the body which would prevent cure.

When radiotherapy is given with the intention to cure, the doses given are quite high, and the side-effects (see below) may be correspondingly more severe. The total course of radiotherapy treatment may be quite long, i.e. from three to six weeks.

Palliative treatment

This is perhaps the more common use of radiotherapy, when a realistic cure is not possible. It can be very effective at controlling cancers and relieving distressing symptoms, giving much improved quality of life.

Tumours can often cause discomfort or pain if they press on a bone or nerve. By giving radiotherapy to shrink the tumour, this can be quickly, and sometimes dramatically relieved. Similarly, if the growth of a tumour is causing a blockage, for example in the gullet, making swallowing difficult, or in the lung, making it difficult to breathe, radiotherapy can open up these passages again. Very much lower doses of radiation are used in these circumstances, and therefore side-effects are much less severe and sometimes non-existent. And because the doses are low, the treatment can often be repeated if the same problem develops again.

Total body irradiation

People who are having a bone marrow or stem cell transplant (see p.62–68) for a cancer of the bone marrow such as leukaemia, may be given a low dose of radiation to the whole body. This has the effect of permanently destroying the bone marrow, which is extremely sensitive to radiation. This is only possible because the bone marrow is to be replaced with the transplant.

Having radiotherapy

Radiotherapy is only given in cancer treatment centres, as it requires multi-million pound equipment, housed in specially built buildings. For many this usually means that some travel is necessary, often over some distance, to get to the nearest centre.

The specialist doctor who prescribes and plans treatment is called a radiotherapist, or clinical oncologist. Radiographers are

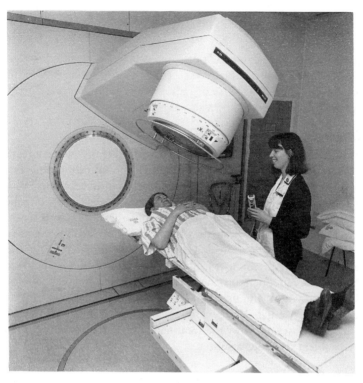

Figure 3 Radiotherapy.

the health professionals who actually give the treatment day to day.

External radiotherapy

External radiotherapy is usually given as an out-patient procedure. This means that it is not necessary to stay in hospital overnight, but instead to come in for a session every day, usually Monday to Friday, with a break at weekends. If the radiotherapy is being given with curative intent, the whole course of treatment may continue over several weeks (perhaps between three and six). If it is given to control symptoms, the course is likely to be much shorter, and may consist of only one or a few sessions. Some hospitals have hostels where people can stay during their radiotherapy treatment, or it may be possible to arrange to stay locally, if the journey is too far or too tiring to make every day of the week. Radiotherapy itself may cause fatigue (see 'side-effects' p.53), and this can be compounded if the travelling to and from the hospital is also long and tiring.

Planning the treatment

The radiotherapist needs a very accurate picture of the tumour before she or he can plan the treatment, and a number of X-rays and scans may be needed. If treatment is being given with the hope of curing the cancer, one or more very detailed planning sessions will then be needed, to ensure that the radiation beam is aimed with pinpoint accuracy at the tumour, and that as little normal tissue as possible is affected. This planning is often done by using a 'simulator' machine—essentially a mock-up of a radiotherapy machine—which uses rays of light to show the doctor exactly where the radiation beam will go.

The area to be treated will often be marked during the planning session, to make sure that all the treatments are given to precisely the same place. The marks may be made on the skin in ink (and if so instructions will be given about not washing these off until the treatment course if finished), or with tiny permanent tattoo marks under the skin.

When radiotherapy is being given to alleviate symptoms, it may not be necessary for the radiotherapist to plan the treatment so meticulously. The much lower doses of radiation used mean that there is also much less risk of damage to any normal tissue in the area treated.

When it is particulary important to keep one part of the body absolutely still, for example, when treatment is given to the head and neck, a perspex mould may be made of that part, to hold it exactly in the same position each time. First, a plaster of paris cast is made of the head, with holes for the mouth and nose, and the perspex mould is then made from the cast. Marks can be drawn on the mask, rather than on the skin, and the mask is fixed to the couch used during treatment.

Having external beam treatment

Radiotherapy is completely painless and while the machine is on, the patient has to lie very still. The radiographers position the person being treated on a couch under the machine, with pillows or wedges to ensure that they are placed as securely and comfortably as possible. The radiographers then leave the room and close the door, so that they are not exposed to radiation while the machine is working. They watch through closed-circuit TV, however, and two-way communication is possible via an intercom. Normally the treatment only lasts a few minutes.

It can be a frightening experience at first, as the radiotherapy machines are very large, and during the few minutes of treatment the patient is alone. However, people become accustomed to the machines, the noise they make, and get to know the staff who are treating them, so that visits should become less stressful. Most departments play relaxing music of the patient's choice during treatments.

Internal radiotherapy

This is given for particular cancers, particularly of the cervix, womb, and breast. For breast cancer, plastic tubes are inserted into the breast, under general anaesthetic, and radioactive wires are threaded through these. For cancers of the womb and cervix, a radioactive source is placed into the neck of the womb, under general anaesthetic.

Internal radioactive sources are left in place only for a few days, but during that time it is necessary to stay in hospital, usually in a separate room. To protect the hospital staff from the cumulative effect of repeated exposure to radiation, the doctors and nurses will only come in for short periods. Short visits from family and friends (though not children, nor pregnant women who may be particularly vulnerable) may be allowed, or they may be able to talk from outside the room.

Once the radioactive sources are removed from the body, all traces of radioactivity disappear.

A more sophisticated way of giving internal radiotherapy to the cervix and womb is by using a machine called an afterloader which can safely store and transfer the radioactive source. Applicators are inserted into the neck of the womb and attached to the machine. When it is switched on, radioactive sources are passed into the applicators; when it is switched off, they are pulled back into the machine. This allows visitors and staff to come and see the person being treated without risk of exposure to radiation, and it also allows a more accurate dose to be given to the area.

With radioactive iodine, similar precautions are taken. After injection it is necessary to stay in hospital for several days, in a separate room, until the radiation dose has worn down to a safe level. Before leaving hospital, clothes and belongings will be checked with a Geiger counter to ensure that they have not been contaminated.

Side-effects of radiotherapy

Generally, the side-effects depend on what part of the body is being treated. Now that radiotherapy is more sophisticated and accurate, side-effects tend to be less severe, and improved methods of treating and alleviating side-effects are available. The radiotherapist should discuss these before treatment begins, giving an idea of what side-effects to expect, and what can be done to prevent or treat them. If other symptoms develop during the course of treatment, they should always be mentioned to the staff, as there is almost always something that can be done to help.

Tiredness is a common side-effect of radiotherapy, whether it is given externally or internally, and to whatever part of the body. This can be quite debilitating, and continue for several weeks after the course of treatment has finished. Rest before and after treatment is essential. Tiredness is to be expected; it is not a sign that the disease has come back or is getting worse.

When radiotherapy is given to an internal organ, there is usually very little effect on the skin. However, if the treatment is being given to the skin itself, or to tissue near the skin, it may turn red and can be quite sore, like sunburn. Advice is usually given before treatment begins about how to care for the skin so as to minimize any reactions. Some radiotherapy departments advise against washing the area at all during the course of treatment; others suggest the gentle use of lukewarm water and then patting the area dry very gently. Most departments do not recommend the use of lotions, talc, deodorants, or perfumed soaps, as these can all make the skin sore. If the skin does become sore and red, cream or lotion should not be applied to the area, unless it has been specifically recommended by the radiotherapist or the radiographer. If the skin reactions are severe, the radiotherapist may decide to postpone further sessions of treatment until the skin has healed. Any effects of radiotherapy on the skin will go once the treatment has finished, usually within two to four weeks.

If radiotherapy is given to a large area and the bone marrow is affected, the levels of red cells, white cells, and platelets in the blood may be temporarily lowered. This is more likely to happen if chemotherapy is also being given with radiotherapy and it is unusual for it to be severe, but occasionally people may require blood transfusions, antibiotics (if the white cells are affected), or platelets to prevent bleeding.

Hair loss only occurs in the area that has been irradiated. Thus, radiotherapy to the head will probably cause some hair loss, and chest, armpit, and pubic hair will be lost if those areas are treated. This hair loss is only temporary, and the hair will start to grow back again once the treatment is finished, usually within two to three months. However, most people who have radiotherapy do not lose their hair.

Specific side-effects

Radiotherapy to the brain will cause hair loss and tiredness. If very high doses are given with the intention of curing a brain tumour, the hair loss may be permanent.

Radiotherapy to the head and neck can cause a sore, dry mouth and difficulty in swallowing. The mouth and throat may be susceptible to infections, especially thrush, and mouthwashes and anti-thrush medicines will be given to try to prevent this. If the mouth is very sore, painkillers can help—they are usually only necessary for a few days, but some people need to continue with painkillers for several weeks. A dry mouth and a loss of taste may persist for quite a long time after treatment has finished—in some cases, many months.

Hair is lost from the area that is being treated but usually starts to regrow some months after treatment is finished.

Radiotherapy to the chest usually causes very few symptoms other than occasional tiredness but may cause difficulty in swallowing if the oesophagus is irradiated. It may be necessary to have a very soft diet for a while, until swallowing becomes easier again. Here, too, anti-thrush medicine may be given to prevent infection, and painkillers if the throat is sore. Some people develop an unpleasant metallic taste in the mouth which may continue throughout the treatment and some time afterwards.

If a large area of the lung is being treated, this may cause shortness of breath, which is usually temporary (a few weeks only). It may be treated with steroids and antibiotics, to cure any inflammation. However, rarely it is caused by permanent scarring of the lung, and in this case, the breathlessness is also permanent.

Radiotherapy to the abdomen can cause diarrhoea, nausea, and occasionally mild vomiting, loss of appetite and, rarely, weight loss. Very effective anti-sickness medicines can be given if necessary, and it may be necessary to consult a dietician to make sure that enough nourishment is being consumed, perhaps supplementing with nutritious drinks.

Radiotherapy to the pelvis can also cause nausea, diarrhoea, and loss of appetite. Since the bowel may be affected it is essential to ensure an adequate diet.

If the radiotherapy affects the bladder, this causes a mild inflammation so that the bladder wall is sensitized. This causes a need to urinate frequently and a burning sensation when urine is passed. This is usually only temporary, lasting just a few days, and it can be easily treated with medicines to make the urine more alkaline.

When women have radiotherapy to the pelvis it is almost impossible to avoid irradiating the ovaries. This will bring on the menopause in women who have not yet had a natural menopause, and will mean they can no longer bear children. For most women, hormone replacement therapy can be given to counteract troublesome menopausal symptoms, but the psychological effects of losing their fertility may be hard to come to terms with, and support and counselling should always be offered.

Caesium implants in the cervix can cause narrowing (stenosis) of the vagina which develops over time after treatment has finished. This can be prevented by regularly dilating the vagina, either with regular sexual intercourse or by using vaginal dilators and a lubricant.

For men, radiotherapy to the pelvic area has no direct effect on their sex lives, although men often lose interest in sex as a result of feeling ill and tired.

Conclusion

Radiotherapy is one of the key treatments for cancer. Its role in the treatment of different cancers, and the best ways of using it in combined modalities of treatment, are constantly being researched and assessed. Modern techniques of giving treatment are now highly sophisticated, enabling the most accurate possible targeting of the rays on the tumour, while sparing the surrounding tissue as much as possible. While radiotherapy can occasionally cause long-term side-effects, these are usually treatable; most side-effects of the treatment resolve quickly once the course of treatment has ended.

Chemotherapy

What is chemotherapy?

Chemotherapy is the major type of drug treatment for cancer. There are a number of other treatments which are also, strictly speaking, chemical treatments, for example hormonal therapy, immunotherapy, but the term chemotherapy has come to mean specifically treatment with cytotoxic drugs—i.e. drugs which act by destroying cancer cells. This chapter discusses cytotoxic treatment; hormonal treatments such as tamoxifen and immunotherapies such as interferon and interleukin-2 are discussed in the sections on tumours for which these treatments are used.

Cytotoxic drugs work by interfering with the process by which cancer cells divide to produce new cells. The drugs are introduced into the bloodstream and circulate round the body. This has a great advantage over other treatments for cancer. It is often not possible to eliminate all cancer cells with surgery or radiotherapy, which are local treatments—i.e. they treat one particular area of the body only. This is because a few cells may break away from the primary tumour and travel in the bloodstream, coming to lodge in some other part of the body where they start to grow as secondary tumours, or metastases. Because chemotherapy drugs take this same route, they can reach these rogue cells and secondary tumours in whatever part of the body they lie.

The first chemical treatment which worked on this principle was the use of antibiotics for infections. Antibiotics destroy the bacteria that cause infection wherever they are in the body. Bacteria, however, are very different in their nature from the normal cells of the body, so antibiotic drugs can be formulated which interfere with the bacteria without causing any damage to normal cells. Cancer cells, however, are only subtly different from normal cells. They have lost the mechanism which controls their growth and reproduction, but in other respects most of the chemical processes of both kinds of cell are the same. So drugs which interfere with cancer cells tend to do some damage to normal cells too.

Although cancer cells tend to be thought of as virulent, they are in fact relatively defective, compared with the body's normal cells, and are less able to repair themselves. The way in which chemotherapy is given takes advantage of this defect; treatment is usually given over a period of one to a few days, and then there is a break of several weeks. During this time the body's normal cells repair themselves while the cancer cells often repair themselves very little. Further cycles of drug treatment are used to continue to deplete the cancer cells while allowing the normal cells to repair themselves again and again as necessary.

It is possible to cure some types of cancer with chemotherapy alone. However, at this time, the majority of cancers cannot be cured by chemotherapy and in this situation the treatment is given to control and shrink the cancer and to relieve symptoms on its own. The main reason why chemotherapy does not cure the majority of cancers is either that the cells become resistant to the drugs, or they are partially or completely resistant to the drugs from the start. For example, if a cancer is 99 per cent sensitive to drugs, chemotherapy could eliminate 99 per cent of the cancer but have no effect whatever on the remaining 1 per cent which would continue to grow. Resistance to drugs and the incomplete killing of all cancer cells are the biggest stumbling block to improving the cure rates and this area is the focus of much research.

Cancer cells become resistant to a drug by developing biochemical processes which overcome the damage caused by the drug. One way to tackle this is to give several different drugs, each of which damages the cancer cells in a different way. It is more difficult for the cells to develop several different protective mechanisms at the same time, so the chances of permanently destroying them are greater. This method of giving chemotherapy has significantly increased cure rates for some cancers but unfortunately cancer cells can sometimes become resistant to several drugs at the same time.

Another way to overcome resistance is to give very much higher doses of chemotherapy. The problem with this is that such high doses also cause a lot of damage to normal cells, especially those of the bone marrow, where the blood is manufactured. These high doses are only possible if 'rescue' by means of a bone marrow or stem cell transplant can be done (see p.62–68).

The bigger a tumour is, the more likely it is to be resistant to drugs. Therefore, if a primary cancer has been removed by surgery and there is a high risk that small clumps of cancer cells have already spread to other parts of the body, rather than wait for a relapse, when the cancer would be harder to treat, chemotherapy can be given immediately after the operation to 'mop up' any cancer cells left behind. This is called 'adjuvant' chemotherapy. Its use is now common in the treatment of many cancers, for example, breast cancer, bowel cancer, and children's cancers and has led to increased cure rates. The use of adjuvant chemotherapy is discussed in detail in the sections on the tumours for which it is relevant.

How is chemotherapy given?

Chemotherapy can be given by mouth, more commonly into a vein (intravenously), and occasionally by injection under the skin (subcutaneously). The intention is to get the active anti-cancer agents into the bloodstream so that they circulate in order to reach the cancer cells wherever they are. Occasionally chemotherapy is given directly into specific areas of the body, for example into the fluid around the brain, or directly into the abdomen. In this case the aim is to give a high concentration of the drug to the area.

The easiest method of giving chemotherapy is by mouth, as a tablet or liquid. This enables chemotherapy to be taken at home, without a nurse or doctor in attendance. However, this is a less reliable method than by injection, as one cannot be sure that the same amount of the drug has been absorbed with each dose.

The commonest method is to give chemotherapy into a vein, either as an injection or, more frequently, via a drip. This usually means that the treatment has to be given in hospital either as an out-patient or an in-patient. Often, people who are having a long course of treatment have a Hickman line (or central line) inserted. This is a length of plastic tube which is tunnelled under the skin of the chest and into the big vein in the chest. One end remains outside the body and drugs can be injected through it. The line is put in under anaesthetic and remains in for the length of the treatment; it should not cause any discomfort.

Each dose of chemotherapy is given over a period of between one and a few days and is repeated at intervals of between one and four weeks (depending on the schedule), for a total of four to eight cycles. Sometimes, low doses are given continuously, via a small portable pump connected to a Hickman line. The pump trickles the drugs into the body over several weeks or even months. The patient can continue with everyday activities, carrying the pump attached to a belt or in a handbag.

Short-term side-effects

Chemotherapy can cause a number of different side-effects and in the past these were often very severe, making the experience of treatment often very unpleasant and notoriously hard to bear. Today, chemotherapy has changed out of all recognition; new drugs cause fewer side-effects, while often also being more effective than the older drugs, and far better methods are available to alleviate and prevent side-effects.

The three most common side-effects of drug treatment are nausea and vomiting, hair loss, and effects on the bone marrow.

- *Nausea and vomiting* used to be the most distressing side-effects of chemotherapy. One of the most important modern developments in cancer treatment has been the development of very effective anti-sickness drugs (anti-emetics). These can often eliminate sickness, and it is now unusual for someone having chemotherapy to be uncontrollably sick. As chemotherapy drugs have been improved too, and often cause less sickness, many people now go through a course of chemotherapy without any sickness at all.

- *Hair loss* occurs with some, but not all, chemotherapy drugs. It can be no more than a slight loss and thinning of the hair, but it can be total, sometimes including hair on the rest of the body as well as the head. This can be a distressing feature of cancer treatment, as people find it hard to adjust to this change in their appearance and it can seem a very public sign of their illness. Many people wear wigs, or cover their heads with scarves or hats. The hair loss is only temporary and the hair will always grow back once the treatment is finished, at its normal rate. With a few chemotherapy drugs, it is possible to reduce the amount of hair lost by cooling the scalp for half an hour during treatment, which reduces the damage to the hair roots by the drug.

- *Effects on the bone marrow* occur because the cells of the bone marrow are particularly sensitive to chemotherapy drugs. The bone marrow produces the cells which form the blood; red cells, white cells, and platelets. When the numbers of these cells are depressed because of damage from cytotoxic drugs a number of different side-effects may be experienced: tiredness and weakness from anaemia caused by lack of red cells; susceptibility to infections caused by low levels of white cells; and bleeding and bruising caused by insufficient numbers of platelets.

All these side-effects can be controlled to a significant degree, and blood tests will be taken at regular intervals during chemotherapy treatment to check on the levels of the cells and to anticipate and treat any problems. Anaemia is treated with blood transfusions. If the white cells are low, or likely to be low, injections of growth factors can be given to boost their number. Platelet transfusions (similar to blood transfusions, but of platelets only) can be given if the platelet count is low. New growth factors are now being developed and it is likely that effective platelet growth factors will be available in the not too distant future, to treat and prevent problems with bleeding due to low platelet counts.

Other short-term side-effects

Diarrhoea is a common side-effect of some, though not all, chemotherapy drugs. It can often be simply and effectively treated with remedies bought over-the-counter from a pharmacy. If it is severe, the chemotherapy may be stopped temporarily, or the dose may be reduced until the problem has resolved.

Fertility. Some chemotherapy drugs can affect men's fertility by decreasing the number of sperm in the semen, leading to the man becoming infertile, sometimes permanently. Chemotherapy can also affect women's ovulation, again leading to temporary or permanent infertility. Questions about fertility, if appropriate, should be discussed with the doctor before the chemotherapy takes place, so that any helpful measures can be taken. For example, a man might want to consider sperm banking, in which samples of his sperm are stored frozen, in case he might want a family later. Storing women's ova is now being tried experimentally, and may become available. People who have become infertile because of treatment may need counselling and emotional support to help them come to terms with this loss.

Women whose treatment causes a permanent menopause can usually be given hormone replacement therapy to counteract the symptoms which may be troublesome.

Sex. There is no reason not to have sex while having chemotherapy treatment, although people may not feel well enough because of other side-effects.

As the effects of chemotherapy on fertility are somewhat uncertain and unpredictable, it is always advisable to use an effective contraceptive during and for a while after treatment, whichever partner is having the treatment, as there is a risk to a child conceived during treatment. Men who are having chemotherapy should also consider wearing a condom, as women have sometimes reported stinging and burning from their partner's semen.

Long-term effects

Some chemotherapy drugs do pose a small risk of causing certain other cancers to develop in the future. This only affects about 1 or 2 per cent of people who receive these treatments, and usually a new cancer does not develop for ten years or more after the original treatment. Not all drugs have this potential, and doctors will avoid using those that do, wherever possible.

Conclusion

Advances in recent years, in the drugs themselves, in methods of delivering the drugs, and in the ways that side-effects can be alleviated, or even prevented in the first place, have made chemotherapy a far less traumatic treatment than it was, even ten years ago. Nowadays, doctors often hear the comment that their patients have found it far easier than they had anticipated. Nevertheless, it is still a stressful and very anxious time, and many people need the support of families and friends, to help them cope and maintain a positive attitude during what can seem like a marathon course of treatment.

Many research studies and clinical trials are going on all the time into new and better methods of giving chemotherapy in almost every cancer. Some of the most exciting results are coming from research into the best ways of combining it with other treatments such as radiotherapy and surgery, to cure, or to prolong life in situations in which this was not possible before.

Bone marrow and stem cell transplants

What are bone marrow and stem cell transplants?

Bone marrow and stem cell transplants are procedures which allow very high doses of cancer treatment, principally chemotherapy but also sometimes radiotherapy, to be given. Because such treatment would destroy the bone marrow permanently, it would not normally be feasible, as the body would lose its vital ability to manufacture the cells in the blood. However, if healthy bone marrow (the substance which manufactures the blood) or stem cells (the primitive cells in the bone marrow which develop into blood cells) can be given back after the treatment, the body can replace the bone marrow and recover its ability to make blood. Bone marrow and stem cell transplants therefore enable high doses of treatment to be given to try and cure a particular cancer, when lower doses would not cure it.

There are two kinds of transplant: allogeneic, which uses someone else's marrow, and autologous, which uses the patient's own bone marrow or stem cells. Autologous transplants are not 'transplants' in the true sense of the word and are sometimes called bone marrow or stem cell support.

Bone marrow transplants are the 'classic' transplants. The aim of removing the bone marrow is to obtain the primitive cells (stem cells) contained within it, which later go on to develop into the various components of the blood. Before any intensive treatment is given, bone marrow is removed from the hip bones of the patient or donor and is then frozen and stored until needed. This collection of bone marrow is called the harvest. Later, after the patient has had treatment with chemotherapy with or without radiotherapy, the bone marrow is given back via a drip, like a blood transfusion. The marrow circulates round the body in the bloodstream, settling eventually in the hollow spaces in the bones, where it starts to grow and begin the process of blood manufacture again.

Very recently, substances called growth factors have been developed. These are proteins which stimulate the production of large numbers of primitive (stem) cells, so that they spill out from the bone marrow into the blood. The use of growth factors means that it is no longer always necessary to removed bone marrow and reinfuse it; the stem cells alone can be collected from the blood. This has many advantages. More stem cells can be harvested and given back with this technique so numbers of cells in the blood recover more quickly which means that the person having a transplant spends less time at risk of infection. It is also easier for the patient to have stem cells collected from the blood than to have bone marrow taken from the bones and a general anaesthetic is not needed.

Stem cells are usually collected after a course of chemotherapy (either during initial treatment, or possibly a one-off dose for this purpose). When chemotherapy is given, the drugs cause the numbers of cells in the blood to drop initially. A few days later, however, the numbers surge, as the body starts to recover. Doctors take advantage of this by injecting growth factors at this point, to maximize the effect and to ensure that as many stem cells as possible spill out into the blood.

At the moment, stem cell transplants are normally only done with the patient's own stem cells and not with a donor's stem cells. Doctors obviously cannot give chemotherapy to someone who does not have cancer, and collections therefore have to be carried out using growth factors alone. Autologous transplants, however, are increasingly done with stem cells rather than the older bone marrow technique and it is likely that this will increase significantly in the near future.

When are bone marrow or stem cell transplants used?

Transplants can be successfully used either for a primary cancer of the bone marrow (for example, leukaemia) or for other cancers when it is felt that very high dose chemotherapy, sometimes with total body irradiation, might increase the chances of cure. Only a very small proportion of people with cancer, however, are suitable for a transplant. The main criteria for suitability are:

- whether the cancer is sensitive to chemotherapy in ordinary doses, and a good response has been achieved already with chemotherapy. If a cancer has not responded to normal treatment with chemotherapy, it almost certainly will not be possible to treat it successfully with higher doses.

- whether, for allogeneic transplants (with marrow from a donor), there is a suitable donor. Bone marrow for transplanting has to be immunologically the same (HLA matched) otherwise it will damage the body of the person receiving the bone marrow. For most people, the most suitable donor is likely to be a sibling—there is a 1 in 4 chance of matching bone marrow from a brother or sister. Identical twins have identical HLA. Occasionally it may be possible to find a suitable unrelated donor through a donor bank.

- whether, for autologous transplants (with the patient's own bone marrow), there is any cancer in the bone marrow. There is obviously no point in giving back cancer cells. If there are tiny amounts of cancer cells in the bone marrow, it may be possible to clean-up (or purge) the stored bone marrow before returning it; these techniques are however still at an experimental stage.

- generally, whether the person who is to have the transplant is fit and well and reasonably young. Autologous transplants are not usually recommended for people over the age of 65; for allogeneic transplants, an upper age limit of 50 is usual. Stem cell transplants, where the risks are somewhat less, may be possible at slightly higher ages.

The transplant process

There are essentially four steps in the transplant process.

1. *The initial treatment of the cancer*, by conventional chemotherapy and/or radiotherapy, to reduce the cancer to as low a level as possible. Ideally, people who are to have a transplant should be in remission at the time (i.e. there should be no detectable cancer), as this gives the best chance that the intensified treatment will be effective. However, it may still be successful if there is a small amount of cancer still present.

2. *The collection of the bone marrow or stem cells from the patient or donor*. To collect bone marrow, the patient or donor is given a general anaesthetic. About 1 litre of bone marrow is withdrawn, through a syringe, from a number of spots over the hip bones and sometimes

the breast bone. This usually requires a short stay in hospital, and the patient may feel quite sore and bruised afterwards and need mild painkillers for a few days.

Stem cells are collected by a technique called haemophoresis and this is done at the time when the number of stem cells that have spilled out into the bloodstream are at their highest, following chemotherapy and injections of growth factor, as explained earlier. For this process, blood is taken from one arm and spun in a centrifuge, which causes the stem cells to separate out. The remaining blood is then returned into the other arm. The whole process takes about 3 to 4 hours and is not painful.

3. *The treatment.* This takes place in hospital and usually lasts about 4 to 5 days and consists of very high doses of chemotherapy and sometimes total body irradiation as well (see p.49, 57–58 for more discussion of these treatments). A single room is usually provided during this stay in hospital, because of an increased susceptibility to infection. Anti-cancer drugs are usually administered through a central or Hickman line (see p.58), which will be put in under anaesthetic. The line will also be used for giving fluids, taking blood samples, and for giving the bone marrow or stem cells in step 4. Anti-emetics are given to prevent nausea and vomiting, and possibly sedatives to make the person feel more comfortable.

4. *Giving back the marrow or stem cells.* The bone marrow or stem cells are given back via a drip into the central line, like a blood transfusion, and will find their way back to the bones. It will be a few weeks, however, before the body starts properly manufacturing blood again, and during this time the patient is very carefully monitored. Low numbers of white cells will make people very vulnerable to infections and regular antibiotics may be given. Even those bacteria in the skin and intestines which are beneficial to healthy people may become harmful and cause infections. Particular care will be taken not to introduce infection from outside and there may be restrictions on visitors to avoid bringing in infection.

Low numbers of red cells will cause anaemia and make the patient feel very tired. Regular blood transfusions may be necessary until the body is manufacturing enough blood for itself. Transfusions of platelets to prevent bruising and bleeding may be required.

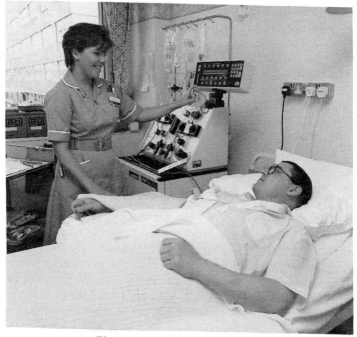

Figure 4 Collecting stem cells.

Even after discharge from hospital, the patient is closely monitored, and will need to return to the hospital for regular checks. Occasionally blood or platelet transfusion continue to be necessary, or changes in medication. It will take up to a year for the immune system to return to normal after a transplant, and the patient may need to return to hospital if they become unwell. Care of health during this period is important, and any symptoms should be reported at once to the hospital where treatment took place (a 24-hour contact telephone number is given on discharge from hospital).

The risks of bone marrow and stem cell transplants

The main risk, for all kinds of transplant, is that of infection which is at its greatest in the two to four week period after the transplant, when the marrow is recovering. Antibiotics will probably be given to prevent as well as treat any infection. In rare instances, however, even with modern antibiotics, an overwhelming and fatal infection may take hold. This is a small, but real, risk of these transplants.

A further serious risk, for allogeneic transplants only, is that of graft-versus-host disease. Even though the donor marrow is matched to that of the recipient, it can only be an exact match in the case of identical twins. There is, therefore, usually some reaction between the cells of the donor (the graft) and those of the patient (the host). Medicines are routinely given to prevent graft-versus-host disease, and the symptoms are usually mild and include skin rashes and diarrhoea and temporary damage to the liver. However, occasionally the disease can be severe and even life-threatening. It can occur up to several months after the transplant.

A further consideration, which needs to be fully discussed if a transplant is on the cards, is the intensity of the treatment. People having a transplant need a high degree of physical and mental stamina. The high doses of chemotherapy and radiotherapy can make people feel ill and can of themselves cause complications. People who are at the upper age limit for transplants, or whose general health is not good, may be at high risk from the treatments themselves.

What conditions are transplants used for?

Bone marrow transplants (almost always allogeneic transplants) have an established role in the treatment of certain leukaemias, in both adults and children, especially when initial treatment has produced a good response but there is a high risk that the leukaemia might return. The high dose chemotherapy with radiotherapy reduces that risk and improves survival rates.

It is not yet proven beyond doubt that transplants increase the cure rate in other conditions, but there are strong suggestions that they do in certain circumstances. Some people with Hodgkin's disease and non-Hodgkin's lymphomas, for example, may benefit. Amongst solid tumours, it has been found that certain kinds of testicular cancers respond to high-dose treatment, and it is now being explored in the treatment of breast cancer in two different contexts: as adjuvant chemotherapy for women who have a high risk of relapse; and for women with advanced disease who have had a good response to chemotherapy and have little disease left. Trials of the use of high dose chemotherapy with bone marrow or stem cell transplants for breast cancer are still on-going and their role has not yet been established.

Conclusion

Bone marrow transplants receive a lot of media coverage and are often interpreted as a wonderful and heroic treatment for all cancers. It is true that their development over the last decade (and the development of stem cell transplants more recently still) has been a tremendously exciting and important advance in cancer treatment. Nevertheless, a certain amount of caution is needed. At this moment, they are only of benefit to a small number of people, in very limited and particular circumstances. Apart from their proven role in the treatment of leukaemia, it is not yet clear what improvement in overall cure and survival rates they make. Over the next few years, as research continues, we will know a great deal more about the role they have to play in the treatment of many more cancers.

8　*Cancers by site of origin*

· ·

Cancer of the head and neck

This group of cancers includes those which start in one of the following: the lip, tongue, mouth, nose or throat (together called the nasopharynx), voice box (larynx), and sinuses. Many possible causative factors have been identified including chewing and smoking tobacco, excessive intake of alcohol, poor dental hygiene, prolonged exposure to hardwood sawdust. In the far east cancers of the nose and throat are thought to be linked to infection by a particular virus but no such association has yet been shown in western Europe. The incidence of cancers of the head and neck has fallen in the UK probably as a result of improvements in oral hygiene, in smoking habits, and industrial ventilation.

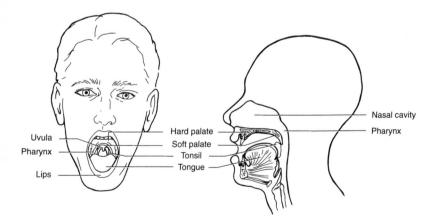

Figure 5　Head and neck.

Presentation

This is a particularly complex area of the body which includes structures with different specialized functions. The most common site for cancers is the larynx followed in decreasing order of frequency by the throat, the tongue, the mouth, the nose and sinuses and finally the lip. Clearly the symptoms will be influenced by the site where the cancer starts. For example a nodule or ulcer which fails to heal situated on the lip or in the mouth or on the tongue is likely to be noticed easily. The same type of nodule or ulcer in the larynx may produce hoarseness of the voice, shortness of breath (because it is narrowing the airway), or less commonly some difficulty in swallowing. Tumours starting in the sinuses may produce swelling and redness of the cheek with or without pain, stuffiness of the nose sometimes with a discharge.

Investigation

If the abnormal area can be seen easily then biopsy should be straightforward and the diagnosis soon be available. For more deep seated problems a general anaesthetic is necessary for this will allow a very careful inspection of the suspect area and also of related structures. For example inspecting the area above the throat and behind the nose and then down to the larynx can be done with a mirror but it is not easy either for the person concerned or the doctor, particularly if a very detailed examination is required. In addition several biopsies may need to be taken.

Apart from the routine tests to check the blood, kidney, and liver function, various X-rays are helpful in looking at the bones and also at soft tissues. The sinuses are usually full of air but if there is swelling of the lining this can show up well on an X-ray. A CT scan may be very useful in showing whether the cancer has spread locally—this is particularly true of some of the deeper areas. As might be imagined this can be very valuable if treatment is to involve surgery or radiotherapy.

Spread of these cancers to distant sites is unusual at the time when people first see their doctor but a chest X-ray is important to exclude spread to the lungs or (since cigarette smoking is implicated in cancers of the larynx *and* lung cancer) a primary cancer of the lung.

Treatment

This depends on precisely where the cancer is, how large it is, and may be influenced by what it looks like under the microscope. Most people are now seen in a 'Joint Clinic' where a head and neck surgeon, a radiotherapist, and a medical oncologist are available to discuss between themselves and with the person the best strategy for dealing with their cancer. The outcome of this may be to proceed to radiotherapy either alone or followed by surgery. Where specialized structures such as the larynx are involved treatment with radiotherapy alone, which preserves function, is favoured if at all possible. In those people who have either a cancer of the larynx, or of the throat above it and where surgery is needed some loss of function may be inevitable. If any form of major surgery is advised as when, for example part of the larynx has to be removed, some speech training will be needed after the operation. The speech therapist has a very important role in helping those who need to regain their speech. Exceptionally the breathing passage may be brought out to the neck (a tracheostomy). In this case speech is made possible by swallowing air and although this sounds unlikely it can be extremely effective, but, like any new technique it requires patience and persistence in learning. Those who have to undergo some form of radical surgery should be reassured that good quality life is usually achievable once confidence is regained. The role of chemotherapy is currently being explored in clinical trials. While this is disappointing in advanced disease there is a suggestion of a possible role around the time of surgery.

Other cancers of the head and neck

These include cancers of the skin (see p.167–172), the salivary glands, and those in and around the eye.

Cancers of the skin may appear as areas of crusting or as ulcers which fail to heal or as small nodules with a pearly surface. These changes are most likely to be seen in someone who has had chronic exposure to sunlight. If there is any doubt it is better to seek medical advice. It is often possible to make a diagnosis by taking scrapings from the lesion and looking at them under a microscope. The nodules with a pearly surface may be found anywhere on the face but also on the ear and are usually proved to be what was called a 'rodent ulcer' (a basal cell carcinoma)—these are true cancers which tend only to spread locally. They can usually be cured by surgery or local radiotherapy. The more serious cancers of the skin are 'squamous cell' cancers—these do spread and so are treated by a wide excision and then often radiotherapy as well. They are regarded as more serious really because they are difficult to control if they recur or if they spread to another site. Further surgery and then chemotherapy are usually advised. There are a number of drugs which are active against these cancers—the best of these are cisplatin, methotrexate, and bleomycin. Although quite good responses may follow their use there is little evidence that survival is improved so that the main emphasis of treatment must be on quality of life. This means that the side-effects of the chemotherapy must be kept to a minimum in order to favour any benefits. Sometimes people needing chemotherapy are in rather a poor nutritional state which may make the side-effects of the treatment particularly hard to circumvent.

Cancers of the salivary glands

There are two groups of salivary glands: the parotids lie in each cheek just in front of the ear and drain into the mouth inside the cheek alongside the teeth of the upper jaw; the submandibular glands lie below the floor of the mouth and drain into the area below the tongue.

Cancers of these glands are rare—occasionally they are involved by lymphoma (see p.173–184). Lymphoma may occur in a gland which has been damaged in a more general illness (an 'auto-immune' disease where the body's very effective defence mechanisms do some damage to otherwise normal tissues). However the more common cancers found in the salivary glands are those which start in the cells of the glands themselves. Cancers of the submandibular glands are very rare indeed, it is the parotid gland in which most salivary gland cancers are found.

Presentation

Usually these cancers present as a slow growing, painless swelling in a cheek. Occasionally the cancer damages one of the main nerves to the face which runs very close to the parotid gland and produces a weakness of the face on that side. This combination of a painless swelling and weakness of the face is very suggestive of a cancer in the parotid gland. Rarely swelling may be noted to one side below the jaw—in this case within the submandibular gland.

Investigation

Although what are generally called routine tests will be carried out (to check that there is no anaemia, gross infection, or inflammation, tests of kidney and liver function and a chest X-ray) the most important test is the examination by the pathologist of all or part of the swelling under the microscope. The surgeon will probably advise that the swelling should be removed and although he may ask for a piece to be examined under the microscope during the operation, to give him some idea of how extensive the surgery should be, it is likely that he will proceed to the removal of the tumour. This avoids the need for a second anaesthetic and clearly a growing lump is better removed. Sometimes this can be quite a difficult procedure particularly as he will want to try to avoid damaging the big nerve to the face. Sometimes, where the cancer has grown around the nerve, this is unavoidable and the consequence is likely to be paralysis of the face on that side. In some people a temporary weakness of the face is present after the operation but clears up spontaneously.

Radiotherapy is frequently given after the operation in order to cut down the risk of the cancer recurring. If the tumour was very small, was almost benign, and had a very well formed capsule around it then radiotherapy may not be necessary. Even with widespread or recurrent disease chemotherapy does not appear helpful.

Prognosis

The outlook after treatment for cancers of the head and neck depends very much on their site, how advanced the cancer is, how completely it can be removed, and also on its appearance under the microscope. Early disease is potentially curable by surgery usually in combination with radiotherapy. In advanced disease surgery, radiotherapy and chemotherapy may be used alone or in combination in an attempt to control the cancer. Overall women appear to have a rather better outlook than men.

Cancers of the eye socket

Most commonly these are cancers which have spread from elsewhere but some very rare cancers may begin in the eye socket and these include tumours of the muscle around the eye (rhabdomyosarcoma); of the nerves (glioma); of cells which circulate in the blood and which are normally found in lymph glands (lymphoma). As might be imagined any swelling in the eye socket can distort the eye. This and watery swelling of the eyelids and distortion of the eye itself are the most common ways in which these cancers may declare themselves.

Investigations

X-rays of the eye socket can show a great deal of useful detail, but a CT scan or magnetic resonance scan can show the precise location of any tumour and the degree to which it has spread. Ultrasound can given useful preliminary information. Rhabdomyosarcoma is principally seen in childhood. It may spread to the bone marrow so that bone marrow examination (see p.34) is an important examination.

Treatment

Radiotherapy is the treatment of choice for most of the cancers which have spread to the eye from elsewhere (metastases) and the outlook is that for the primary cancer. It is usually the primary treatment for localized lymphoma which tends to be very sensitive. For other cancers surgery may be the primary treament with or without radiotherapy.

The treatment for rhabdomyosarcoma is now well standardized but may involve very specialized radiotherapy techniques followed by chemotherapy using combinations of drugs. The five year survival for rhabdomyosarcoma within specialist centres has now risen to around 75 per cent.

Cancers of the eye

Although rare, the commonest tumour to start in the eye is melanoma which may first come to attention either at a routine eye examination or because of disturbances of vision. It is rare to find evidence of spread when people first present but spread, particularly to the liver, is common some years later. Because of this the initial tests may include an ultrasound examination of the liver. Previously the whole eye was removed but now, if the melanoma is small and causing no particular problems many eye surgeons will recommend conserving the eye for as long as possible. Local treatment can be given using a laser, by radiotherapy, or cryosurgery. If the eye becomes painful, the pressure within the eye rises or there are signs to suggest the cancer is becoming more extensive then removal of the eye is likely to be recommended.

Cancers of the thyroid gland

These cancers are more common in women than men. Some may occur in a thyroid gland which may have had a prolonged abnormality, others may occur in someone who had radiotherapy given in the neck area for some quite unrelated reason. In women there is an initial peak incidence between the ages of 30 and 40 and then, as in men, a steadily increasing incidence from about 50 onwards. There are several very different kinds of thyroid cancer, the commonest is called 'papillary' because of its appearance under the microscope. This accounts for very nearly two thirds of all thyroid cancers and is three times more common in women than in men. 'Follicular' cancers are much less common and are the kind found particularly in people who have had a goitre for a very long time. 'Medullary' cancer may occur in different members of the same family and may form part of a 'multiple endocrine neoplasia' (MEN) syndrome in which other rare cancers may be found. These other cancers may involve the adrenal gland (there are two and each lies over the upper pole of a kidney). 'Anaplastic' thyroid cancer is the kind most commonly found in elderly people.

Presentation

Most commonly this is as a painless swelling in the root of the neck. If the swelling is large this may make breathing noisy because of narrowing of the breathing passage. Occasionally the cancer may grow into a nerve called the recurrent laryngeal nerve which supplies the vocal cords, the damage it causes to this nerve may make the

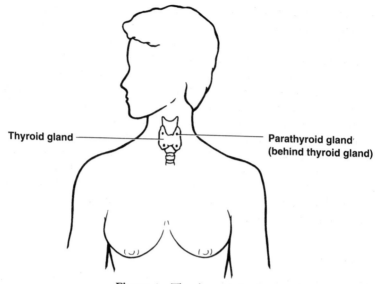

Figure 6   The thyroid gland.

voice sound hoarse. People with medullary cancer of the thyroid which is part of the multiple endocrine neoplasia syndrome (MEN) may sometimes have hormone problems caused by their overproduction by one of the affected glands. This might cause high blood pressure, diabetes-like symptoms (great thirst, passing volumes of urine, and feeling generally unwell) or problems caused by high calcium in the blood (depression, constipation, occasionally tetany).

Investigation

Blood tests are needed to measure thyroid hormones and the hormones which drive the thyroid (these are produced in the pituitary gland within the brain). If MEN is suspected other blood tests will be needed to see whether there are abnormalities which might support this diagnosis. Isotope scans of the thyroid involve an injection of radioactive iodine (I^{131}); this is taken up by the thyroid gland and then using a special camera the thyroid gland is scanned (i.e. moved over the gland in a regular way level by level). Whereas the normal gland is working to take up the iodine the cancerous area contains cells which are too primitive to work so 'cold' areas are seen. Of course a cyst (that is a pocket of fluid) will also be cold and indeed only about 20 per cent of cold areas turn out to be cancers. It is sometimes helpful to draw out some of the fluid and cells from a cold area to look at under the microscope— this may be enough to give a diagnosis, but if there is doubt an operation will be necessary. Before an operation takes place an ultrasound examination of the thyroid, a CT scan, a chest X-ray, and a bone scan will probably have been done to determine whether any distant spread can be found. Lymphomas can sometimes start in the thyroid gland and since these can be very widespread it is normal to do a CT scan of the chest and abdomen, a bone marrow examination and special blood tests for evidence of lymphoma in the blood. Only when a very full assessment has been made can treatment be considered.

Treatment

Apart from lymphoma of the thyroid where chemotherapy alone, or occasionally with radiotherapy, is the treatment of choice the primary treatment of thyroid cancer is surgery—the usual procedure is a near complete removal of the thyroid in order to minimize the risk of leaving behind a small focus of cancer. Any localized abnormal tissues which might contain cancer are also removed (it is helpful to look at this under the microscope to see whether it is in fact involved by the cancer). In the case of medullary and anaplastic cancers the surgeon may aim to remove some of the nearby glands in case some of the cancer cells have spilled over into them. Since follicular and papillary cancer both take up radioactive iodine this can be given in high doses as treatment after surgery with the intention of killing any remaining focus of the cancer. Before this is done a further I^{131} scan will be done to determine whether any obvious cancer remains. Treatment with I^{131} is given as a drink but because the dose of radiation is fairly high it is necessary to stay in hospital until the levels of radiation in the urine and stools are low. It is a little intimidating to have such attention given to one's waste products but since the results of this form of treatment are so good it is worth bearing with the inconvenience.

If distant disease is found, and this is more likely with medullary and anaplastic cancer, local control with radiotherapy is attempted. Chemotherapy has not been found to be particularly useful.

Prognosis

The type of cancer, its extent, the sex of the person, and the age at diagnosis all influence the likely outcome. A tumour which is made up of cells which look fairly like normal thyroid cells, occurring in someone under 40 years of age, is likely to be cured. About three quarters of those with papillary and follicular cancers which have not spread outside the thyroid are alive at ten years, and even those which are more widespread can do very well. The comparable figure for medullary cancers is more than a third while for anaplastic cancers the long-term outlook is less encouraging.

Lymphomas of the thyroid tend to respond well to combination chemotherapy but some patients are elderly and tolerate chemotherapy poorly. About half can expect long-term survival.

Brain tumours

There are two very distinct kinds of brain tumours, primary and secondary brain tumours, and it is important to be clear about the difference between them. Primary brain tumours, which are uncommon, start in the tissue of the brain itself, and do not very often metastasize and spread. Secondary brain tumours, which are much more common, are tumours which have started elsewhere in the body (for example the lungs and the breast) and have spread to form new tumours in the brain. The reason this distinction is so important is that secondary cancers in the brain may respond to different treatment from primary brain cancers. Thus a tumour in the brain caused by a primary breast cancer is likely to be responsive to treatment for breast cancer.

Overall, the incidence of primary brain tumours is very low. They mainly occur in older people, but there is a significant incidence in children and adolescents. Tumours in the brain account for quite a high proportion of all childhood cancers (though it must be remembered that childhood cancers are themselves rare).

There are a number of kinds of primary brain tumour. In adults, the commonest (about 50 per cent) are astrocytomas, also called gliomas. These vary in the degree of aggressiveness they manifest, and are usually divided into: low grade astrocytomas, which are slow growing; intermediate grade anaplastic astrocytomas; and high grade astrocytomas, or glioblastoma multiformae, which grow most rapidly.

The next most common kind of brain tumour is the meningioma, which affects the membrane covering the brain (the meninges). These tumours are almost always benign (that is, they rarely show signs of malignant change). However, benign tumours can cause severe problems as their growth causes them to press on vital structures in the brain. Other adult tumours, also almost always benign, are pituitary adenomas (which affect the pituitary gland) and neurilemomas (which affect the nerve sheath).

Astrocytomas are the commonest primary brain tumours in children, accounting for about 45 per cent of all such cases. About 20 per cent of brain tumours are medulloblastomas, which most commonly occur in the cerebellum; a further 10 to 20 per cent are craniopharyngiomas, which are generally benign but cause symptoms due to pressure on other parts of the brain.

The reasons why primary brain tumours occur are not known. There is some evidence to show that there may be a genetic factor in the cause of some brain tumours. Other suspected factors include exposure to certain chemicals, a suppressed immune system, and previous exposure of the head to radiation treatment. Obviously, the cause of a secondary brain tumour is always a primary tumour somewhere else in the body. Occasionally, people may not be aware that they have cancer until symptoms of what turns out to be a secondary tumour occur. Once tests have established that the tumour in the brain is indeed a metastasis, not a primary, further tests may be needed to find the primary tumour and to try and treat it.

Presentation

The symptoms of primary and secondary brain tumours are identical. A severe and persistent headache is often the first symptom. This may be made worse by coughing, sneezing, or bending over, and may make sleep difficult, and still be present in the morning. It may often be associated with nausea and vomiting. Frequent bad headaches are a good reason to seek medical advice; it is extremely unlikely that they are caused by a brain tumour, but it is wise not to leave them uninvestigated.

Other symptoms of a brain tumour can include mental confusion, or occasionally personality changes. Depending on which part of the brain is affected, vision, speech, or balance may be disturbed or impaired, and there may be weakness on one side of the body.

Investigations

If a brain tumour is suspected, there will be referral to see a specialist neurologist. The first tests she or he will carry out will be to examine the neurological system. The doctor will look into the eyes with an ophthalmoscope to see whether the optic nerve at the back of the eye is swollen (which may happen when there is increased pressure inside the brain due to the growth of a tumour). Other tests will be done to test the strength of the arms and legs, balance, reflexes, sensation and possibly some mental exercises.

If these tests indicate the possibility of a brain tumour, the next step will be to scan the brain, either with a CT scan of the head (see p.38) or with an MRI scan (see p.40). These techniques build up a picture of the brain which may enable the doctor to see the tumour and any swelling (oedema) around it.

If the scans show a tumour, and there is known to be a primary cancer elsewhere in the body, there will be no need to biopsy the tumour. However, if there is no known primary, it will be necessary to take samples of the tumour itself and examine them under the microscope for a definite diagnosis.

A biopsy from a brain tumour involves a major operation under general anaesthetic. Depending on where the tumour lies, and how difficult the operation, it may be possible to attempt to remove most or all of the tumour during the diagnostic operation. If the tumour is too inaccessible to remove it altogether, then a sample only will be removed for examination. For details of the operation, see below under 'Surgery'.

Treatment

Steroids

As most brain tumours cause swelling in the tissue around them, which is itself the cause of many of the symptoms, steroids are very often used as soon as the diagnosis has been made to reduce the swelling. These drugs act quickly and most people rapidly feel better and many of their symptoms, including weakness in the limbs, improve or even disappear. However, these drugs have no effect on the tumour itself.

Surgery

If it is possible to remove the tumour with surgery, this is the treatment of choice for primary brain tumours. Occasionally surgery may be used for secondary tumours when there is only a single spot in the brain, and there are no metastases anywhere else in the body. Generally, however, surgery is not used for secondary tumours.

The operation is done under general anaesthetic. The head is shaved, and a flap cut in the scalp. The surgeon then removes a piece of bone above the site of the tumour. The tumour, or as much of it as possible, is removed surgically, then a metal or plastic plate is put back, to replace the piece of the skull, and the flap of skin is stitched back over the site.

Depending on the part of the brain that is affected and the tissue that the surgeon has had to go through to reach the tumour, some weakness or impaired brain function, which may be permanent, may inevitably result from this operation. The surgeon will explain what is likely to happen, before the operation.

Radiotherapy

Radiotherapy is frequently used after surgery, to treat any malignant tissue that was impossible to remove surgically, or to mop up any tiny collections of cancer cells that may have been left. Very careful planning of radiotherapy to the head is necessary, so that the radiographer can aim the beam of radiation with absolute accuracy. It may be necessary to wear a perspex mask during the treatment (see p.51), to keep the head still and to ensure that the treatment is always given to exactly the same spot. For a technique called stereotactic radiotherapy, in which doses of radiation are very accurately aimed at the head, from several different angles, to achieve maximum damage to the tumour with the least possible damage to normal tissue, it may be necessary to have the head held in a frame.

Another approach is brachytherapy, or internal radiotherapy, which allows a high dose of radiation to be delivered to the tumour itself with minimal damage to surrounding tissue. For this, radioactive substances are placed directly in the tumour. Special techniques, as for stereotactic treatment, are used to pinpoint the exact placing of the radioactive sources. Internal radiotherapy is sometimes used as well as external beam treatment.

For secondary tumours in the brain, usually a smaller dose of radiotherapy is given to the whole head, and such extremely careful planning is not usually needed.

Radiotherapy to the head causes hair loss over a period of a few weeks. The hair will grow back again after treatment is finished. There are few other side-effects.

Chemotherapy

A number of drugs are used to treat certain primary brain tumours, particularly intermediate and high grade astrocytomas and medullo-blastoma. The aim of drug treatment is to shrink and control the tumour, not to cure it. Chemotherapy is sometimes given as well as radiotherapy, as it seems to improve the results of radiotherapy. Hormonal treatment, such as tamoxifen (see p.97) may also be given with chemotherapy, as it seems to make chemotherapy more effective.

Prognosis

A proportion of people with low grade astrocytomas can be cured with combined treatment of surgery and radiotherapy. For many people with brain tumours, however, treatment is given with the aim of alleviating symptoms and prolonging life by controlling the cancer for as long as possible.

Lung cancer

Causes

Cancer of the lung is the one cancer for which an incontrovertible cause has been established. Since the 1950s, it has been known that smoking, particularly cigarette smoking, is by far the most common cause of lung cancer (accounting for over 90 per cent of cases).

Before the beginning of the twentieth century, lung cancer was a very rare disease, and the pattern of incidence during this century has mirrored social trends in smoking. As lung cancer may take several decades to develop, the peak period of cigarette smoking amongst men in the 1930s and 1940s was reflected in the incidence of lung cancer in men peaking in the 1950s, 1960s and 1970s, while the incidence among women (among whom smoking was not generally common until the Second World War and after) is still increasing in older age groups. Although there is now a small decline in incidence among men, it is still the commonest male cancer, and the second commonest for women, after breast cancer, although in some areas it has now become more common than breast cancer, for women. And as smoking is increasing among women, especially young women, the increase in female lung cancer is likely to continue. Overall, lung cancer accounts for about one quarter of all cancer deaths.

Clear links have also been established to show that the longer someone has been smoking, and the more cigarettes they smoke, the higher the risk of getting lung cancer. Low-tar and filtered cigarettes reduce the risk somewhat, as it is thought to be the tar content of cigarettes which contains carcinogens (although some smokers may take more puffs of each cigarette to compensate for the milder yield). Smoking other forms of tobacco, such as cigars and pipe tobacco, carries a much lower risk than cigarettes.

Passive smoking—inhaling other people's cigarette smoke—has been associated with an increased risk of lung cancer. Non-smokers who live with someone who smokes, and people who work in smoke-filled environments (such as pubs, clubs, and restaurants) have a slightly increased risk, although this is still much smaller than the risk of actually smoking themselves. It has nevertheless been recognized as a risk by many organizations, which has led to the banning of smoking in many public places, offices, public transport, etc. in many countries.

A number of other carcinogens are known to cause lung cancer. Working with asbestos and uranium mining are both high-risk industries. Radon gas, which is a naturally occurring gas, can reach high levels in some geographical areas and has been associated with lung cancer.

Prevention

The single most effective way of reducing the risk of lung cancer is to stop smoking. Ten to 15 years later, an ex-smoker's risk of getting lung cancer is similar to that of someone who has never smoked.

There is some evidence to show that vitamin A (beta-carotene) which is found in green and yellow vegetables may have a protective effect.

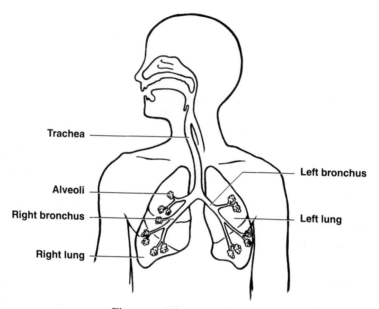

Figure 7   The respiratory tree.

Presentation

The most usual symptoms of lung cancer are:

- a cough that does not get better, even after treatment with antibiotics

- coughing blood

- shortness of breath

- pain in the chest

- general symptoms of weakness and weight loss.

Investigations

Following a general examination, the first test is usually a chest X-ray. While this cannot make a definite diagnosis of lung cancer, it can show up suspicious patches on the lungs and prompt further investigations.

Sputum cytology, in which a sample of phlegm is examined under a microscope, may be enough to give a definite diagnosis and to identify what type of lung cancer is present. If not, a bronchoscopy will usually be performed. This procedure involves passing a thin flexible tube down the throat into the airways of the lung. The doctor can look through the bronchoscope to check for abnormalities and take samples of cells for examination in the laboratory. A bronchoscopy is usually done under local anaesthetic.

If surgery is being considered, the doctor may need to examine the local lymph nodes in the chest, and so a mediastinoscopy may be performed. This is done under general anaesthetic and involves a small tube being passed into the chest through a cut at the base of the neck. Samples of cells and lymph nodes will be taken for examination.

Other tests, such as a CT scan of the chest and abdomen, an ultrasound scan of the liver, and bone scans may be done to find out whether there has been any spread of the disease.

The types of lung cancer

There are four main types of lung cancer:

- squamous cell cancer—the commonest type, accounting for about 50 per cent of cases. It occurs mainly in the cells that line the airways.

- adenocarcinoma, which accounts for about 20 per cent of cases, and develops from the cells that produce mucus.

- large cell carcinoma, so called from the large, rounded shape of the cancer cells. This accounts for about 10 per cent of cases.
  These three types of cancer are collectively known as 'non-small-cell lung cancers' as their progression and treatment differs from the fourth type:

- small cell or 'oat cell' carcinoma, so called from the distinctive shape of the cells which resemble oat grains. This cancer accounts for about 20 per cent of cases.

Treatment

Treatment decisions depend on the type of lung cancer. Non-small-cell cancers, if diagnosed at an early stage, are less likely than small-cell cancers to have spread to other parts of the body. Surgery is, therefore, the preferred first line treatment if investigations show no sign of spread. Small-cell cancers, however, have usually spread by the time of diagnosis, so surgery is less likely to be effective. However, these cancers are very sensitive to chemotherapy and radiotherapy.

Non-small-cell cancers

The first question to be determined is whether surgery is possible. If the tumour is in the lung itself, and the lymph glands are not involved, and if the person is fit enough, then surgery to remove part or all of the affected lung gives a reasonable chance of cure. However, only about 25 per cent of people with these cancers are eligible. Others are not suitable, either because the disease has already spread, or because their unaffected lung is not sufficiently healthy to sustain them after the operation, or they are otherwise unfit to have the operation.

For someone who is not fit, but who has a small tumour confined to the lung, radical radiotherapy to the tumour can occasionally cure the cancer and will, more often, shrink the tumour so that symptoms can be alleviated. It is not known whether this treatment actually prolongs life. Radiotherapy is often kept in reserve for when symptoms get very troublesome because of its very helpful palliative effect.

Chemotherapy in advanced disease has been show to shrink the cancer in a proportion of patients, and to prolong life somewhat. The aim is to control symptoms and give better quality of life.

More recently, chemotherapy has been used before surgery and radiotherapy (neo-adjuvant chemotherapy). There is now some evidence to suggest that this may improve survival to some extent. Further studies are now going on to find out how best to use this combination of treatments to maximum benefit.

Small-cell cancers

Surgery is very rarely used to treat these cancers as they have usually spread to other parts of the body before the cancer is diagnosed.

Chemotherapy is usually the treatment of choice. It has been shown to prolong survival, and, in a very small proportion of patients, to provide a cure. A combination of drugs is usually used, and their side-effects are comparatively mild, and can be well controlled, although loss of hair is almost always a side-effect.

Radiotherapy, given after chemotherapy, also has a useful role, as these cancers are very sensitive to this treatment. It is particularly useful if the disease has not spread beyond the chest. It also has a palliative role to play in shrinking the tumours if they are causing symptoms such as pain.

Prognosis

A small minority of people with lung cancer are cured, mainly by surgery. About 25 per cent of people who are able to have surgical resection of the lung are cured. A small number of people with small cell tumours also appear to be cured. Most deaths from this disease occur within a year or two of diagnosis. However, many people's lives can be prolonged by appropriate treatment with surgery, radiotherapy, and chemotherapy, and their symptoms can be controlled, giving a reasonable quality of life.

While much work is being done to improve treatments for lung cancer, it is clear that health education campaigns to prevent people taking up smoking and to help them give it up play perhaps the most vital part in the battle against lung cancer.

Rare lung tumours

Mesothelioma

This is not strictly a cancer of the lung, but of the pleura (the membrane which lines the lungs). It has been known for at least 60 years that this disease is largely caused by exposure to asbestos. There are a significant number of people, however, who get mesothelioma, who apparently have not been exposed to asbestos; however, this disease takes a very long time to develop (usually 30 to 40 years) and it is often difficult to establish with certainty whether or not someone has been in contact with this substance, particularly as it was used in an enormous number of ways because of its fireproof qualities, for example in buildings, vehicle brake linings, ironing boards.

Exposure to asbestos is known also to increase the risk of other lung cancers, particularly in people who smoke.

Mesothelioma causes the lining of the lungs to thicken and fluid to develop over the lung. This causes shortness of breath, which is often the first symptom. The diagnosis is made with a biopsy (either a needle biopsy under local anaesthetic, or an open biopsy under a general anaesthetic), but it can sometimes be difficult to establish a definite diagnosis even by examination of the cells under a microscope.

If mesothelioma is discovered early, it may very occasionally be possible to remove the lining of the lungs with surgery, and thereby to eliminate the disease. Usually, however, cure is not possible, although such an operation may be done to relieve breathlessness. Chemotherapy and radiotherapy can also be used to shrink and control the cancer, but their roles remain experimental.

Bronchoalveolar carcinoma (alveolar cell carcinoma)

This is a type of adenocarcinoma of the lung which often presents as several spots of cancer on both lungs. On X-ray it can sometimes be confused with pneumonia. Surgery and radiotherapy are not practical as treatments, because of the large number of areas to be treated. Chemotherapy can play a helpful role in controlling the cancers for some time.

Carcinoid tumours

These can occur as primary cancers of the lung. When they do they behave very similarly to the more common carcinoid tumours of the gastro-intestinal tract, see p.134.

Breast cancer

Cancer of the breast is the most common cancer in women and probably the most feared. Every year nearly 25 000 new cases are diagnosed, and every year approximately 15 000 women die of breast cancer—more women than die of any other cancer. It is the commonest single cause of death in all women aged 35 to 54. The risk of getting breast cancer has been calculated as 1 in 12, for all women, and for certain groups of women this risk increases substantially as we shall see.

But the fear that breast cancer holds for many women does not lie only in statistics about risk and mortality but in the fact that breast cancer attacks a part of the body that for most women is very important to her feelings about herself as a woman, and treatment almost always involves surgery to the breast. For this reason there has been an enormous growth in recent years of different organizations to support women who have breast cancer—from specialist nurse counsellors working in hospitals, to organizations such as Breast Cancer Care, to local support groups made up of women who have been through the same experience.

Treatments too have changed. Improved surgical techniques and the use of radiotherapy mean that most women now have a choice about the kind of operation they have, and whether or not they have reconstructive surgery afterwards. Chemotherapy and hormone therapies, alone or in combination, too are improving the chances that a woman will not have a recurrence. Better diagnostic techniques and the provision of a national screening programme are ensuring that cancers of the breast are found earlier, when the chance of cure is better.

Causes of breast cancer

1. Age

The risk of getting breast cancer increases substantially the older a woman is. It is very rare in women under 20, but the incidence increases steeply from the age of 35 onwards and figures show an incidence of 300 cases per 100 000 in women aged 85 and over.

2. Hormonal factors

It has been firmly established that there is a relationship between hormone levels, particularly oestrogen, and the development of breast cancer. Many breast cancer cells contain proteins called oestrogen receptors. It appears that oestrogen can be taken up by these receptors into the cell where it encourages the cell to grow.

Any individual woman's 'hormonal history' is an important factor in determining her risk of developing breast cancer. A woman who started menstruating very young, and/or had the menopause very late, is at greater risk because her body will have been exposed to the fluctuating levels of oestrogen associated with the menstrual cycle for longer than average. The same is true of women who have had no children, or who have had their first child late in life. Early childbearing, the number of children a woman has had, and breastfeeding all decrease the risk—by increasing the amount of time she has been out of the cycle of menstruation.

Early versions of the contraceptive pill, which contained quite high doses of oestrogen, have been slightly implicated in the development of breast cancer. Newer formulations of the pill, in which lower dosages of oestrogen were combined with another hormone, progesterone, are very unlikely to contribute to breast cancer. Hormone replacement therapy, which replaces oestrogen in postmenopausal women to reverse the effects of the menopause, may pose a very small risk, but one which most people believe is far outweighed by the benefits. The risks of prolonged use of both the pill and HRT are still being evaluated.

3. Genetic factors

It has been shown that there is an hereditary factor which increases the risk of breast cancer in some women. Women who have one or more first-degree relatives (their mother or sister) with breast cancer are at slightly higher risk themselves; if their relative's cancer occurred premenopausally, or affected both breasts, the risk is somewhat greater.

4. Dietary factors

Breast cancer is a disease of the western developed world. More than half of all cases of breast cancer in the world occur in North America and Europe. There is a strong possibility that there may be links between some features of the lifestyle of the developed world, and the development of cancer.

Direct correlations between diet and the development of breast cancer have not been made, but there is a strong suspicion that a diet high in animal fats (meat and milk products) may promote breast cancer, possibly by raising the levels of oestrogen circulating in the body. People who are obese, and who have a very high calorie diet are at higher risk, probably because animal fats are a substantial part of their intake.

5. Other factors

There is no evidence to show that damage to the breast (e.g. caused by knocking it) causes breast cancer. If a woman has a history of benign breast disease (mastitis, benign breast lumps, or cysts) she may have a slightly increased risk of contracting malignant breast disease.

Presentation

Most breast cancers manifest themselves first as a small lump in the breast. Very often this is first noticed by the woman herself. Most breast lumps are benign but they should always be checked out by a doctor as soon as they are discovered, as the smaller a breast tumour is when diagnosed, the better the chance of a successful cure. For very small tumours the cure rate is 90 per cent; for tumours less than 1 cm in diameter, the cure rate is 70–80 per cent. The outlook is less good the larger the tumour is, and if the lymph glands in the armpit have been affected.

Breast awareness/self-examination

As most breast lumps are first picked up by women themselves it is important that every woman should be aware of the normal changes that take place in her breast, for example at different stages of the menstrual cycle. By looking at and feeling her breasts while, for example, bathing, showering, or dressing, she will be able to get to know what is normal for her, and will be alerted when she notices anything out of the ordinary.

Women can also learn a more thorough technique for examining their breasts, using the tips of the fingers to feel round the breast and up into the armpit. This procedure was until recently the one promoted by health professionals, but many women felt uncomfortable about doing it, or guilty at not doing it, and official opinion now is that 'being aware' is just as effective in detecting lumps early.

Signs to watch out for:

- lump or thickening in the breast

- change in outline or shape of the breast

- puckering or dimpling of the skin on the breast

- flaking of the skin on the breast

- discharge from the nipple

- thickening or lump on the nipple

- inverted nipple

- swelling of upper arm or armpit

- unusual pain or discomfort in the breast.

The presence of these symptoms, or concern at anything unusual in or on the breast, are indications to seek prompt medical advice.

Breast screening (mammography)

Mammography is a technique for examining the breasts by X-ray. It can be used to detect very tiny cancers, before they are large enough to be felt—when the chance of cure is highest. Because the breast tissue in women under 35 is very dense, mammography is not very successful in detecting cancers in this group. It is however very effective in older women. Since 1988, there has been, in the UK, a national screening programme to offer all women between the ages of 50 and 64 a mammogram once every three years. It is estimated that by the year 2000, there will be 25 per cent fewer deaths from breast cancer among the age group eligible for screening.

During the mammogram, the breast is pressed between two plates (which some women find uncomfortable) and exposed to a very small dose of X-rays. There have been some fears that this exposure itself could lead to an increased risk of breast cancer. However,

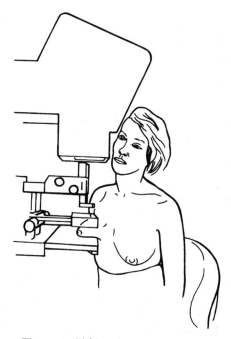

Figure 8   Taking a mammogram.

as the dose of radiation is extremely small, the risk is very tiny indeed, and far outweighed by the benefits of early detection of breast cancer.

Women who are considered to be particularly at risk of developing breast cancer may be advised to have more regular mammograms, or to have them at a younger age. For women under 35 who are at risk, ultrasound scanning can be used instead to examine the breasts.

Investigations

Women who have a suspicious lump or other symptoms of breast cancer will be referred by their GP to a specialist and will probably undergo most or all of the following investigations to confirm the diagnosis.

Mammogram

Even if the suspect lump was detected at a routine mammogram, she will probably have another which will focus more specifically on the area of concern. Younger women may have an ultrasound scan of the breasts instead.

Needle aspiration

A very fine needle will be inserted into the lump and a sample of cells extracted into a syringe for examination in the laboratory. This is a very quick and simple procedure.

Needle biopsy

If a needle aspiration is not possible, a slightly larger needle may be used to extract a small piece of tissue from the lump. This test is done under local anaesthetic. The sample is then sent for examination in the laboratory.

Excision biopsy

In most cases, the doctor will know whether the diagnosis of breast cancer is confirmed or not from these tests. Occasionally it may be necessary to remove the lump and send it for examination. This operation will be done under general anaesthetic and will probably mean a short stay in hospital.

Further tests

If the previous tests have confirmed that a woman has breast cancer, she may undergo further investigations, such as an ultrasound scan of the liver, or a bone scan, to see whether the disease has spread. As well as detecting breast cancer, or confirming the diagnosis, the results of these tests enable the doctor to decide what 'stage' the breast cancer is at. Because different treatments, or combinations of treatment, are appropriate for breast cancer at different stages, decisions about treatment cannot be made until the stage is established.

Stage 1. The tumour measures under 2 cm in diameter. The lymph nodes in the armpit are not affected. The cancer has not spread elsewhere in the body.

Stage 2. The tumour measures between 2 and 5 cm in diameter, or the lymph nodes are affected, or both, but the cancer has not spread further.

Stage 3. The tumour is larger than 5 cm in diameter. The lymph nodes are usually affected, but there has been no further spread.

Stage 4. The tumour is any size. The lymph nodes are usually affected and the cancer has spread to other parts of the body. This is secondary breast cancer.

Treatment

Surgery

Almost all women who have breast cancer have surgery to remove their cancer. In the past, the operation used was a full radical mastectomy, which removed the breast entirely as well as the muscles in the chest wall and the glands in the armpit. It was found that if only the tumour was removed, little spots of cancer were left behind and the cancer eventually came back. The radical mastectomy therefore gave the best chance of eradicating all the cancer.

Nowadays, however, radiotherapy, chemotherapy, and hormone

therapy can be used to deal with any remaining cancer cells left behind after surgery. Such drastic surgery is now rarely if ever necessary, and for many women there is now a choice as to the type of operation she is to have. It has been shown that there is no difference in the survival rates of those women who have mastectomies as compared to those who choose a lesser operation.

Lumpectomy

This operation removes the breast lump and the tissue surrounding it. It removes the least amount of breast tissue of any of these operations, and once the wound has healed, the appearance of the breast is usually good, which has obvious psychological benefits to the woman. This operation is always backed up by radiotherapy to the breast to deal with any tiny spots of cancer that may remain.

Segmentectomy or quadrantectomy

This operation is similar to a lumpectomy but it removes a larger amount of tissue and therefore the results are more noticeable. This too is always followed up by radiotherapy.

Mastectomy

For some women, a mastectomy is the most appropriate treatment, for example those whose cancer is just on or below the nipple, or those who have a large tumour in a small breast. Nowadays the operation is likely to be a simple mastectomy (removal of the breast tissue) or a modified radical mastectomy (removal of the breast tissue together with a small muscle from the chest wall). These operations may be followed by radiotherapy to the chest and armpit if it is thought that there is a high risk the cancer will return.

With all these operations the surgeon will usually remove lymph glands from the armpit as well. This is done to check whether any cancer has spread from the breast. Some surgeons will remove all the lymph glands, while others remove only some glands, as a representative sample.

Breast reconstruction

It is now possible for reconstructive surgery to be done at the same time as a mastectomy, or it can be done at a later date. For many women it can be enormously beneficial psychologically to have a breast reconstruction. There are two basic methods of reconstruction. One is to use the body's own muscles (usually a muscle in the back, channelled round into its new position with its blood supply intact); the other is to use an implant. There have been scares about the safety of silicon implants following reports about leakage of silicon and the possibility that this could cause cancer. There have also been worries that an implant, and the hardening of the body's tissues around it, could disguise the growth of a new cancer on the site.

Radiotherapy

Radiotherapy is used frequently after surgery of all kinds for breast cancer. Its purpose is to treat the area of the breast and the armpit (if only some of the lymph glands have been removed) to ensure that all remaining cancer cells have been eradicated. This is especially important after the smaller operations of lumpectomy or segmentectomy; it may not be necessary after a mastectomy.

External beam radiotherapy is normally given as an out-patient, in a course of daily sessions over a few weeks. Internal radiotherapy is given as an in-patient. Women who have external radiotherapy to the breast after their operation may also have internal radiotherapy too, although this is becoming less common. Very occasionally, women may have internal radiotherapy alone.

For internal radiotherapy, narrow tubes (the width of drinking straws) are implanted in the breast, while the woman is under a general anaesthetic, either at the same time as the original surgery or, more commonly, later. Wires containing a radioactive source (usually iridium) are placed in the tubes and left there, usually for 3 to 4 days, during which time she will have to be nursed in a room on her own.

Adjuvant therapy and treatments for advanced breast cancer

Adjuvant therapy is treatment that is given after surgery when there is no definite evidence of spread of the cancer but where there is a strong likelihood of the disease coming back in the future. The reason it may recur is that there may be small clumps of cancer cells (micrometastases) remaining which are too tiny to detect by currently available scans but which later grow and become detectable. Doctors can tell who is more likely to have micrometastases by looking at the appearance of the cancer and the glands under the microscope. People are described as having advanced disease when there is definite evidence of spread to other parts of the body.

It can be seen from this that adjuvant therapy is given to many women after treatment for their primary cancer in order to reduce the risk of the cancer coming back. Both chemotherapy and hormone therapy are used; the kind of treatment a woman has is principally dependent on whether or not she has reached the menopause.

Many of the treatments used as adjuvant therapy are also used for women whose breast cancer has metastasized (i.e. women who have advanced, or secondary, breast cancer). Treatment for metastases will depend on a number of factors, including which part of the body is affected, whether the cancer is oestrogen-receptor positive, whether the women is pre- or postmenopausal, and what kind of treatment she had in the first instance.

Hormone therapy

Hormone treatment is most usually given as adjuvant therapy to postmenopausal women. It has been shown to reduce mortality by about 25 per cent in this group of women. For the treatment of advanced disease, hormonal treatments are generally more effective in controlling metastases in the bone and soft tissues. Hormone treatments are generally very safe to take and, although a few women experience troublesome side-effects, they are rarely serious. Tamoxifen is probably the best known and most common hormone given both as adjuvant therapy for postmenopausal women and as treatment for advanced disease whether or not the woman has had the menopause. It works by preventing oestrogen from being taken up by the oestrogen-receptors inside the cancer cells; it therefore blocks the mechanism by which oestrogen encourages the cell to grow. Artificial forms of progesterone (such as Provera or Megace) work in the same way as breast cancer cells often have receptor sites for progesterone as well as oestrogen.

For women who have not yet had the menopause, stopping the ovaries from functioning (either by an operation to remove them, or by giving them a dose of radiotherapy) will reduce the levels of oestrogen in the body effectively, and this may be done either as adjuvant therapy or as treatment for secondary breast cancer.

However, as these procedures inevitably cause permanent infertility, doctors sometime prefer to use for adjuvant therapy one of a group of drugs which have the same effect, but are reversible. These drugs are known as pituitary downregulators, or LHRH analogues, and they act on the part of the brain called the hypothalamus, stopping it from producing a 'releasing hormone'. Normally this releasing hormone acts on the pituitary gland, stimulating it to produce hormones which in turn act on the ovaries and cause them to produce oestrogen. By interrupting the process, the ovaries are 'switched off' and the levels of oestrogen in the blood fall.

For the treatment of advanced disease, another drug, aminoglutethimide, may be given to postmenopausal women, especially those with metastases in the bones. Although, after the menopause, a woman's ovaries will no longer be producing oestrogen, a certain amount will still be produced in the body's tissues. Aminoglutethimide interferes with this process and therefore prevents this oestrogen production. This treatment is not suitable for premenopausal women as it does not affect production of oestrogen by the ovaries.

Chemotherapy

As adjuvant therapy, chemotherapy is more effective for younger women, who have not yet reached the menopause. Here, the results of chemotherapy mirror those of hormonal therapy in the older age group.

For the treatment of advanced disease, chemotherapy is generally used for metastases in the liver or lungs, and for those women for whom hormonal treatments are no longer effective. Various different chemotherapy regimens are used and drugs are used singly or in combinations. Perhaps the most common combination therapy is CMF (cyclophosphamide, methotrexate, and 5-fluorouracil). If many glands are affected by the disease, a more intensive regimen with adriamycin as a single agent might be used. If more than 10 glands are involved, it may sometimes be possible to give very high doses of chemotherapy followed by a bone marrow or stem cell rescue.

Prognosis

Breast cancer can be cured; the earlier it is detected, the better the prospects for cure. Sixty-four per cent of women are alive at least five years after their diagnosis of breast cancer. But five-year survival rates diminish depending on the stage at which the cancer is diagnosed:

- Stage 1: survival rate 84%

- Stage 2: survival rate 71%

- Stage 3: survival rate 48%

- Stage 4 (metastases): survival rate 18%.

The likelihood of cancer recurring depends on the extent of the disease when it was diagnosed. Some women may experience a local recurrence in or near the operation site, or in the remaining breast tissue after a lumpectomy. More often metastases appear in one or more other parts of the body. The most usual sites for metastases are the lymph nodes, the skin, the bones, the liver, the lungs, and the brain. While secondary cancers cannot usually be cured, they can be very effectively treated and controlled. Many metastases are very slow growing and can be kept in remission for a long time. In addition to the treatments described above, there are many effective drugs and other palliative measures which can ensure that the symptoms caused by breast cancer metastases are well controlled and that women have a good quality of life, sometimes for years. Many women with advanced breast cancer are older, and may well live a normal life expectancy and die of some other cause than their breast cancer.

Rare breast cancers

Paget's disease

This form of breast cancer in women accounts for about 1 per cent of all breast cancers. It presents as an itchy eczema-like rash on the nipple, which may bleed, and biopsy of the nipple will show cancer cells in the skin. In most cases, further examination reveals a tumour in the breast tissue, sometimes some way from the nipple.

The standard treatment is mastectomy, as the involvement of the nipple makes smaller operations difficult. However, recent small studies have shown that an operation to excise the nipple and the underlying cancer, followed by radiotherapy, gives similar results.

Male breast cancer

Men can also get breast cancer, although this is very rare. In the UK there are only approximately 200 cases a year, occurring almost always in men aged over 60 years old. A much higher proportion of male breast cancers (80 per cent) are oestrogen-receptor positive, but in general, breast cancer in men is very similar to the same cancer in women and responds to the same treatments. Randomized trials of treatments specifically for male breast cancer have not been possible, as so few cases occur that meaningful results cannot be obtained. Generally the prognosis for men with breast cancer is similar to that for women.

The most usual symptom is a lump on the breast. Standard treatment is to remove the breast, but local excision followed by radiotherapy is also now used in some cases. Hormone treatment has a useful role, both as adjuvant therapy and for treating advanced disease. In the past, orchidectomy (removal of the testicles) was the most usual way of affecting the body's hormone levels, but nowadays it is much more usual to give synthetic hormones such as tamoxifen, progesterone, anti-androgens, LHRH analogues, and aminoglutethimide. Chemotherapy is used in similar ways as for women's breast cancers, both as adjuvant therapy and for treatment of advanced disease.

Ovarian cancer

Cancer of the ovary is the fifth most common cancer in women; approximately 1 in 55 women develops the disease, and it is more common as a cause of death than other gynaecological cancers. The most common kind of ovarian cancer, epithelial ovarian cancer, accounts for about 90 per cent of all cases of this disease, and is the one discussed here. The remaining 10 per cent of cases are cancers known as germ cell tumours which develop from primitive cells within the ovary (see below, p.104).

Causes

Cancer of the ovary mainly affects older women and is rare in women under 40. There is some relationship with a woman's hormonal history, in that it is more common in women who have not had children while, conversely, women who have had many pregnancies are at less risk. Use of the contraceptive pill significantly reduces a woman's risk of getting ovarian cancer; a woman who takes the pill for more than five years in her twenties reduces her risk by 50 per cent for the rest of her life.

Worldwide, statistics show that ovarian cancer is far more common in the western industrialized world, indicating that there are almost certainly environmental factors at work too. This is confirmed by studies of women who have emigrated from Japan (which has a very low incidence of this cancer) to the USA. Incidence among second generation immigrants begins to rise to match the figures for the American population. However, no clear cut links with any particular environmental risk factor have been established.

Ovarian cancer seems to be associated with breast cancer, in that women who have one of these cancers are at a greater risk of getting the other. And, as with breast cancer, there does seem to be a genetic element in the development of ovarian cancer in some cases although this is far less than for breast cancer. It is very rare for a woman to have two or more close relatives with ovarian cancer but in that event she is at greater risk of getting it herself. Studies have been undertaken to assess the value of screening to detect early ovarian cancers in women whose risk is increased. Such screening consists of a blood test to check the levels of a substance called CA 125, followed by an ultrasound scan of the abdomen. If both the CA 125 levels and the ultrasound scan are abnormal, there may be an increased risk of ovarian cancer. The benefits of ovarian cancer screening are not yet established and it is therefore not widely offered (see p.24).

Presentation

Cancer of the ovary tends not to cause many or any symptoms until it is quite advanced. Those symptoms it does cause tend to be vague and intermittent. The most common is a swelling in the abdomen, caused by a build-up of fluid, called ascites. Sometimes people experience indigestion, nausea, vomiting, or constipation if the tumour starts to block the bowel. It is unusual for ovarian cancer to cause pain or abnormal bleeding.

Investigations

A physical examination of the abdomen will allow the doctor to feel if there is fluid in the abdomen and sometimes a lump can be felt. An internal vaginal examination may also enable the doctor to feel any lump in the pelvis or on the ovary. However, as many women, both pre- and postmenopausally, have benign cysts on their ovaries which can be quite large, any lump will need to be investigated further to check whether it is benign or malignant.

The next test is likely to be an ultrasound scan (see p.38) or a CT scan (see p.38) to see whether the ovaries look enlarged or in any way abnormal. These scans also provide a picture of the inside of the abdomen, the liver, and the pelvis, so that these areas can be checked for any spread of the disease. Blood tests to check for raised levels of CA 125 (see above) may also be done.

If these tests indicate a strong possibility that a tumour is present, and if there is fluid in the abdomen, a firm diagnosis can be made by drawing off a sample of this fluid, using a fine needle, for examination under a microscope to see if it contains cancer cells. A local anaesthetic is used to numb the skin before this procedure. If no fluid is present, the only way to make a definite diagnosis is to remove the lump surgically, and examine the tissue under the microscope. This is usually done during an operation called a laparotomy, which involves a vertical incision in the abdomen, under general anaesthetic. The same operation is used as the first part of the treatment of the ovarian cancer.

Treatment

Surgery

Surgery is normally the first treatment for cancer of the ovary. It is usually necessary to perform a hysterectomy, removing the uterus (womb); both ovaries; the fallopian tubes which descend from the ovaries to the uterus; and the abdominal fat pad. At the same time, the surgeon explores the whole abdominal cavity to remove any signs of malignant tissue elsewhere. If the bowel shows signs of cancer, it may be necessary to remove the affected piece and rejoin the two ends.

This examination of the abdomen is an extremely specialized form of surgery, and it is important that it is performed by a surgeon who is an expert in gynaecological cancer. Research has shown that even if the disease cannot be completely excised by surgery, and some small patches remain, the subsequent response to treatment is much better the more disease is removed. Sometimes surgeons may need to perform a second operation, some time after the original surgery. The purpose of this 'second look' is usually to see whether the disease has responded to treatment, and to help doctors decide whether or not further treatment should be given.

It can be very distressing to women to have a hysterectomy. For those women who are premenopausal, it brings on an early menopause, with possible symptoms such as hot flushes, dry skin, dryness of the vagina, and depression. It can also be very difficult to come to terms with the ending of their reproductive life. For women who have reached the menopause, a hysterectomy can still be a blow to their sense of themselves as women. All these factors may have profound effects on the emotional wellbeing of women, at a time when they are also having to come to terms with having cancer. It is therefore most important that emotional support and counselling are available before and after the operation, to help women through this difficult time.

Chemotherapy

Ovarian cancer is sensitive to chemotherapy. This treatment is sometimes given after surgery to deal with any tiny pockets of disease that have not been removed at the time of the operation. It is also used to treat disease that has recurred or is advanced.

Many different drug regimens are used. The most important and effective drugs are those derived from platinum. When these drugs were first used they had many distressing side-effects, particularly nausea and vomiting. Newer versions of these drugs, however, have been developed which are much better tolerated and cause fewer side-effects and modern anti-sickness drugs (anti-emetics) are also very effective in controlling nausea and vomiting.

In most cases of ovarian cancer, the disease does not spread beyond the abdominal cavity. Recently, a new technique has been developed which allows drugs to be delivered straight into the abdominal cavity via a thin plastic tube passed through the abdominal wall. This allows higher concentrations of the chemotherapy drugs to be used.

Recent research has shown that a drug derived from the bark of the yew tree, taxol, can significantly affect ovarian tumours, and doctors are now investigating ways of using this drug to best advantage.

Radiotherapy

Radiotherapy does not play an important role in the treatment of ovarian cancer nowadays. As the cancer can involve the whole abdominal cavity, the whole abdomen has to be irradiated, which places severe limits on the amount of radiotherapy that can be given. Some studies have shown that radiotherapy can be helpful in destroying microscopic patches of cancer left behind after surgery. However most doctors feel that both the immediate side-effects (nausea, vomiting, diarrhoea) and later complications such as bowel and bladder obstruction, make this treatment less desirable than chemotherapy, which is usually more effective.

Prognosis

When ovarian cancer is detected at an early stage, surgery on its own, or followed by chemotherapy, can often cure it. When the disease is more advanced, cure can still sometimes be achieved with chemotherapy, but in a much smaller number of people. For most of those with advanced disease, however, the aim of chemotherapy treatment is to control the cancer and prolong good quality life.

Rare tumours of the ovaries

Germ cell tumours

Germ cell tumours represent 2 to 3 per cent of all ovarian tumours and are very similar to testicular tumours (see p.155–160). They occur more often in young women. There are three main types: endodermal sinus tumours, teratomas, and dysgerminomas. The first two are very similar to testicular teratomas and the principles of treatment are also similar. They are rapidly growing and aggressive. In the early stages they may be treated by surgery alone, or otherwise by chemotherapy based on cisplatinum in combination with other drugs such as etoposide and bleomycin. As with testicular teratomas, the prognosis for these tumours is very good, and many are cured even in advanced stages.

Dysgerminomas are similar to testicular seminomas. They are very sensitive to radiation, and radiotherapy was, in the past, the standard treatment. However, radiotherapy to the ovaries stops them functioning permanently. If the cancer is at a very early stage, and affects only one ovary, surgery to remove the ovary can cure the cancer while leaving the other ovary unaffected. Recently, good results have been achieved with chemotherapy, without compromising fertility.

Granulosa cell tumours

These are slow-growing tumours composed of cells which have the ability to produce oestrogen. They occur predominantly in premenopausal women. Treatment is usually by surgery, sometimes followed by radiotherapy if it is not possible to remove the tumour completely. They are also chemosensitive, and treatment with cisplatinum can sometimes give complete remission. As these tumours grow very slowly, if they do recur, it is often many years after the first occurrence.

Mixed mullerian tumours

These can occur as primary tumours of the ovaries. When they do, they behave in a similar way to the more common mixed mullerian tumours of the uterus, see p.116.

Fallopian tube carcinomas

These cancers behave in a very similar way to ovarian tumours. Treatment is by surgery in the first instance (using the same procedures as for ovarian cancer), and chemotherapy has a useful role in the treatment of advanced disease.

Cancer of the cervix

One of the greatest breakthroughs in cancer prevention was the invention of the smear, or Pap test, which can detect precancerous changes in the cells of the cervix (the lower part, or neck of the womb). It is a simple, painless, and relatively cheap test and it has enabled widespread screening to be introduced. Women can be screened at regular intervals so that such changes can be identified and treated when necessary. Studies from a number of countries have shown that the incidence of cervical cancer can be dramatically reduced if a screening programme is introduced and the opportunity for screening is taken up by a large proportion of eligible women.

Early identification of abnormalities means that action can be taken to treat them long before there is any danger they might develop into a cancer, and those women can be carefully followed-up over the years to ensure that no further abnormalities develop.

The need for action to reduce the incidence of this cancer is illustrated by the fact that it is the eighth most common cancer in women in the western world, and worldwide is the second commonest female cancer (in developing countries it is the most common). And while mortality rates are decreasing overall, rates for younger women in their thirties are increasing.

In the United States, it is common for the test to be performed annually. In the United Kingdom, government guidelines recommend that every woman between the ages of 20 and 64 who has ever been sexually active should have a smear test every five years, and most doctors recommend an interval of three years as being preferable.

During the smear test, a doctor or nurse gently scrapes the cervix with a specially shaped wooden spatula to remove some cells for examination under a microscope. The term for any changes or abnormalities in these cells is cervical intra-epithelial neoplasia (CIN) and they are coded CIN 1, 2, or 3 according to whether they are early, moderate, or severe. These changes are not cancerous, and many would never go on to develop into cancers, although some will develop into cancer if they are not treated. Most cervical cancers take many years to develop from the early stages of abnormality.

The major distinction between precancerous changes and cancer is whether the changes are only in the superficial layers of the cervix (in which case they are precancerous) or they have penetrated into the deeper layers of the cervix (in which case they are cancerous). Precancerous changes to the cells of the cervix can be very effectively treated by a number of different methods: cryotherapy (freezing the cells); diathermy (burning the cells); laser therapy (using laser light to destroy the cells); or cone biopsy (surgical removal of the inner part of the cervix). All these methods are equally effective and the cure rate is close to 100 per cent.

Causes

A number of different factors contribute to the development of cervical cancer. There is a clear relationship between a woman's history of

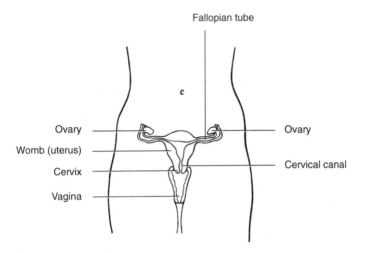

Figure 9 Ovaries, cervix, and uterus.

sexual activity and her risk of developing precancerous changes or cervical cancer: the more partners she has had, and the more partners her partners have had (i.e. the wider the network of sexual contacts), the higher the risk for any individual woman. Women who first had sex at a young age are also more at risk. It appears that some factor transmitted during sex is responsible for the development of many cases, and this is confirmed by the fact that using barrier contraception offers some protection.

Infection with some varieties of a virus known as the human papilloma virus (wart virus), which is sexually transmitted, is thought likely to be one factor in the development of this cancer. However, most people who contract this virus do not get cervical cancer, so there are plainly many other unknown factors.

It used to be thought that taking the contraceptive pill might slightly increase the risk of cervical cancer. It is now believed that the pill itself is not a causative factor, but the fact that women who take the pill are less likely also to use a barrier contraceptive.

Smoking doubles a woman's risk of getting cervical cancer, whatever her sexual history. It is thought that some product of smoking, when absorbed into the bloodstream from the lungs, reduces the body's immunity to other cancer-causing factors.

Many women who get cervical cancer blame themselves or their partners for their illness, because of its link with sexual activity. In fact, this is only one of the many factors leading to the development of this disease, and only a very small proportion of women with the known risk factors develop the disease. It is therefore unreasonable for any woman to blame herself or her partner for getting this disease.

Presentation

Many cases of cervical cancer are diagnosed by a routine smear test before a woman has symptoms. The commonest symptom is vaginal bleeding between periods, or postmenopausally, especially after intercourse. Some women experience pain on intercourse, although generally pain is not a symptom unless the cancer is advanced. Some women may have an unpleasant smelling discharge from the vagina. All these symptoms are even more common with benign conditions such as cervical erosion, but medical advice should be sought if any of these symptoms occur so that the reasons can be investigated.

Investigations

The doctor will normally examine the cervix, gently inserting a speculum to keep the vaginal walls open. This should be painless. Sometimes an area of abnormality will be visible to the eye. The doctor will do a smear test at the same time. If the smear shows minor abnormalities, which will probably revert without treatment, the woman will probably be recommended to have another smear in six months time. If the smear shows more serious changes, the next test is likely to be a colposcopy.

A colposcopy allows the doctor to look at the cervix in greater detail, using an instrument called a colposcope, which also shines a light onto the cervix for greater visibility. For this test, too, a speculum will be used to hold the vaginal walls open. A solution may be painted onto the cervix to make the abnormal areas show up more clearly, and a sample of cells (a biopsy) can be taken for examination. This test is usually done in a hospital out-patient clinic. If the whole area of abnormality cannot be seen with the colposcope, a surgical procedure called a cone biopsy will be carried out, under a general anaesthetic, which may entail a short stay in hospital. The surgeon will remove a small, cone-shaped section of the cervix for examination under the microscope. From this, the doctor will know whether the abnormality is a precancerous change, or a definite diagnosis of cervical cancer.

If these tests confirm the diagnosis of cancer, further investigations may be done to see if the disease has spread. A CT scan of the abdomen and pelvis (see p.38) may be done to give a picture of the size and position of the cancer, and to see whether the local lymph glands have been involved. Magnetic resonance imaging (MRI), another form of scanning (see p.40), is being evaluated at the present time, to see if it can give a more accurate picture.

The doctor may want to perform an examination under anaesthetic, which allows him or her to examine the vagina and cervix thoroughly and to asess the extent of the disease, without causing discomfort. A dilatation and curettage (D and C) may be done at the same time. For this, a small probe is inserted into the womb to scrape the lining. Cells from the lining can also be examined under the microscope.

If treatment with surgery is being considered, a further test called an intravenous urogram may be required (IVU or IVP). For this test, a dye which shows up on X-ray is injected into a vein in the arm. The dye travels in the bloodstream to the kidneys, and an X-ray is then taken. Any changes or abnormalities in the kidneys or urinary system are highlighted on the X-ray screen by the dye.

Treatment

This section deals only with treatment for cancer of the cervix. Precancerous changes to the cells of the cervix are treated (if treatment is necessary) by the methods listed on p.106.

Surgery

Surgery is the usual treatment for cancer of the cervix. The standard operation is a hysterectomy—removal of the womb—together with the nearby lymph nodes. It is not usually necessary to remove the ovaries, and this means that younger premenopausal women do not have a surgically induced menopause. If it is necessary to remove the ovaries in premenopausal women, hormone replacement therapy can be given to prevent menopausal symptoms. Occasionally, for young women with only slight invasion of the cervix and who want to have children, a cone biopsy may be done as treatment.

A hysterectomy is a major operation, and recovery may take a while. It is important to avoid strenuous physical activity or lifting heavy objects for several months after the operation. After the operation sexual intercourse should be avoided for about six weeks, to allow the scars to heal.

Many women find that they need more time before they are ready to resume their sex life after this operation. It can be very distressing to have a hysterectomy and many women find it difficult to come to terms with the loss of a part of themselves which may be intimately connected with their sense of themselves as women. Emotional support and counselling before and after the operation should be available to any woman who needs them, so that her emotional wellbeing is looked after as much as her physical recovery.

Radiotherapy

In the early stages of cervical cancer, radiotherapy is as effective as surgery, but the side-effects are greater and always include loss of ovarian function. For this reason, surgery is the treatment of choice at this stage. If the cancer has spread beyond the cervix, however, and is therefore not curable with surgery alone, radiotherapy is the preferred treatment. Radiotherapy may also be used after surgery, if there is a high risk that the disease might come back, for example if the lymph glands have been affected.

Usually a combination of external and internal radiotherapy is given to ensure effective treatment. Internal treatment is given by inserting one or more applicators, like a tampon, into the cervix while under a general anaesthetic. A radioactive source, usually caesium 137, is inserted into the applicators and is kept there, usually for one or two days. During this time it is necessary to stay in bed, probably in an isolation ward with lead screens round the bed, to protect medical staff and visitors from the radioactivity. Once the radioactive implant and the applicators have been removed, the radioactivity disappears.

The side-effects of radiotherapy to the pelvis include nausea, vomiting, tiredness, diarrhoea, and sometimes painful urination. All these can, however, be well controlled and even prevented with drugs.

Radiotherapy can sometimes cause a narrowing of the vagina, which can make sexual intercourse uncomfortable or painful. Oestrogen creams, and the use of a dilator or regular intercourse can improve this condition. Women who have had internal radiotherapy have a very slight increased risk of infection and should contact their doctor immediately if they develop heavy bleeding, or a high temperature after treatment.

Long term, the most significant effect is that the ovaries are always damaged, which will bring on the menopause in younger women. Hormone replacement therapy can be given to ease the symptoms, such as hot flushes, anxiety, and depression. In a small minority of cases, some women experience narrowing or constriction of the bowel as a result of radiotherapy to the pelvis.

Chemotherapy

Chemotherapy is used in various situations for women with cervical cancer. Women who are suitable for treatment with radiotherapy but are thought to be at high risk of relapse are sometimes given chemotherapy before the radiotherapy, in order to shrink the cancer and give a better chance that the radiotherapy will provide a cure. Another group of women who benefit from chemotherapy are those whose disease cannot be treated with radiotherapy, either because the cancer has spread to other parts of the body, or because they have relapsed after receiving maximum amounts of radiotherapy previously. Chemotherapy is given to shrink and control the disease and relieve symptoms, but it cannot provide a cure.

Various combinations of chemotherapy drugs are used for cervical cancer, mostly based on platinum. Sickness from these drugs used to be very severe and hard to tolerate, but modern anti-sickness drugs are now available which are very effective at controlling nausea and vomiting.

Prognosis

When cervical cancer is detected at an early stage, the outlook is very good and a great many women are cured by surgery alone. If the cancer is too far advanced for surgery but is not widespread throughout the body, radiotherapy can cure a significant proportion of women and prolong a good quality life in others. When the cancer is more advanced, chemotherapy has a useful role in controlling the disease, but is not usually able to provide a cure.

The benefits of detecting this cancer at an early stage are unarguable. In the UK, the screening programme has only just begun to have an impact on the overall mortality figures. Greater efforts to target those women who are not taking up invitations to be screened, better follow-up of abnormal results, and a wider diffusion of health education messages regarding smoking and sexual behaviour are needed to improve this situation.

Cancer of the uterus

Cancer of the endometrium, the body of the uterus, is the commonest cancer of the female reproductive organs; however, it is the least common cause of death among these cancers, due to the fact that it is usually detected at an early stage, when it is very amenable to treatment. Endometrial cancer mainly affects older women between the ages of 50 and 64; it is less common in women under 50.

Causes

There are a number of factors which may contribute to a woman's chance of getting endometrial cancer, although no definite causes have been identified. It is thought that the risk is somewhat increased for women who have never had children, women who are overweight, and those who are diabetic.

Hormonal treatments seem to have an effect on the risk, although the evidence seems somewhat contradictory. A substantial reduction in risk (perhaps as much as 50 per cent) seems to be provided by use of the contraceptive pill. This protective effect seems to be maintained for many years after taking the pill. However, the use of hormone replacement therapy consisting of oestrogen on its own, after the menopause, seems to increase the risk slightly. Nowadays, hormone replacement almost always consists of a combined oestrogen and progesterone tablet. The addition of progesterone seems to counteract the increase in risk provided by the oestrogen. As with the contraceptive pill, most women are recommended to take a break from the therapy once a month, during which time they will menstruate. The use of tamoxifen, for the treatment of breast and some other cancers, may also very slightly increase the risk of developing the disease. However, this increase is so very slight that the benefits of taking tamoxifen far outweigh the risks.

Presentation

Cancer of the uterus usually manifests itself at a very early stage, which allows for prompt treatment and a very good chance of complete cure. The most common symptom is vaginal bleeding. For women who have had their menopause, any vaginal bleeding is abnormal and should be brought to the attention of a doctor; women who are still having periods should consult a doctor if they have bleeding between periods. There are many other causes of irregular vaginal bleeding which are usually benign, but it should always be investigated by a doctor. Occasionally, if the cancer is advanced, pain may also be a symptom.

Investigations

The first test the doctor will do will be an internal examination to feel the uterus and vagina for abnormalities, and to take a cervical smear (see p.106). Though this test is usually used to detect cancer of the cervix, it may also pick up cells shed from the body of the womb which can be examined under the microscope for cancerous changes. If the results of the smear arouse suspicion of cancer, a dilatation and curettage will probably be performed. This procedure is usually carried out under a general anaesthetic. While the patient is anaesthetized, the doctor can stretch the cervix and insert an instrument into the uterus to remove samples from the lining. Examination of these samples under a microscope will give a definite diagnosis.

If cancer is confirmed, a CT scan (see p.38) may be performed, to give a clear picture of the site of the tumour, and to show whether any of the local lymph glands are enlarged, indicating that they may have been affected by the cancer. In some centres, a scan using magnetic resonance imaging (MRI) may be done instead. Its use for diagnostic tests in endometrial cancer is still under evaluation.

Treatment

The great majority of cancers of the uterus are diagnosed at an early stage, and can be cured by surgery alone or with radiotherapy as well, if there is evidence that the cancer has spread. Hormonal therapy is used to control advanced cancers and research into the role of chemotherapy is continuing, but its role is not yet established.

Surgery

Surgical treatment involves a hysterectomy (the removal of the uterus), and usually the removal of the ovaries and the fallopian tubes as well, as these are the organs most likely to be affected by any spread of the disease. The aim is for the surgeon to remove as much of the cancer as possible.

Hysterectomy is almost always a distressing operation for a woman. The removal of the ovaries means that premenopausal women have to deal with the symptoms of menopause brought on by the operation, at the same time as dealing with the fact they have cancer, and with the ending of their reproductive life. Women who have had the menopause may also find it hard to come to terms with the loss of a part of themselves that may be very important to their feelings about themselves. At a time when women feel vulnerable, it is essential that medical staff treat them with sensitivity, and that emotional support and counselling are available to them.

Radiotherapy

If there is any sign that the cancer has spread, or the surgeon is concerned that there may be a high risk of relapse because of microscopic disease, radiotherapy, both externally and internally, will be given to treat the remaining areas of cancer.

External radiotherapy will be given to the pelvis as a series of sessions, probably over a number of weeks. Internal radiotherapy will be given as one session lasting several days.

For this, one or more sealed radioactive sources will be placed in the uterus under anaesthetic. This allows a higher dose of radioactivity to be delivered directly to the tumour inside the uterus. While the radioactive sources are in place accommodation is provided in a separate room, perhaps with lead screens round the bed to protect hospital staff from the radioactivity. Visitors may be restricted. As soon as the sources are removed, the radioactivity disappears.

The side-effects of radiotherapy to the pelvis include nausea, vomiting, tiredness, diarrhoea, and sometimes painful urination. All these can be well controlled and sometimes even prevented with drugs. Sometimes, narrowing of the vagina can occur, which can make sexual intercourse painful and difficult. It is important to keep the vagina open, using dilators, or with regular intercourse, otherwise, it may close permanently. The use of oestrogen creams, and lubricants bought from a chemist, can make intercourse more comfortable and easier.

Hormonal therapy

If the cancer recurs after initial treatment by surgery, with or without radiotherapy, then treatment with hormones may shrink the cancer, control symptoms, and prolong life. The same treatment is used for cancers which are not diagnosed until late, when the disease has spread to other parts of the body.

A number of different hormonal treatments may be used. Endometrial cancer is very sensitive to progesterone, and this is often the first treatment used. Tamoxifen, which has an anti-oestrogen effect, is also effective in controlling the cancer. A group of drugs called LHRH analogues, which work on the brain, preventing it from initiating the production of oestrogen in the body, are also sometimes used.

Hormone treatments are generally very safe to take and have very few side-effects; generally, treatment is in tablet form and is continued over a long period of time.

Chemotherapy

The role of chemotherapy in treating endometrial cancer is still being researched, and it does not play a part in the treatment of primary cancers. In a small proportion of people with advanced cancers, however, it can be useful in shrinking the tumour and relieving symptoms, though it cannot provide a cure.

Prognosis

Up to 90 per cent of cancers of the uterus are cured by surgery, with or without the addition of radiotherapy. As this cancer causes noticeable symptoms so early in its course, treatment can be given promptly before there has been any chance of the cancer's spreading to other parts of the body. For this reason alone, women should be encouraged to report to their doctor any irregular bleeding they may experience.

Rare tumours of the uterus

Mixed mesodermal tumours, also known as mixed mullerian tumours or carcinosarcomas

These tumours, which usually occur in the uterus but may occasionally occur in the ovaries, are composed of two types of cells, carcinoma cells and sarcoma cells (see p.1). They usually affect women aged between 55 and 65. The primary treatment is surgery to remove the tumour. Radiotherapy is sometimes used for recurring tumours, but its role is not established. Chemotherapy based on platinum may be used to shrink the tumour, control symptoms and prolong life, but its role too has yet to be defined.

Leiomyosarcomas

These are tumours of the involuntary muscle of the uterus, and tend to occur in women aged between 45 and 55. The first line of treatment is surgery, and this is often curative, especially in the less aggressive types of this cancer. Radiotherapy and chemotherapy can have a useful role in controlling symptoms, but their role is not yet clearly defined.

Cancer of the oesophagus

The incidence of cancer of the oesophagus varies throughout the world more dramatically than the incidence of any other cancer. It is most common in China, Central Asia, Central and South America, and certain parts of South Africa, but even within one country the incidence can vary enormously between regions; in China, it ranges from 140 per 100 000 in the north to 1.4 per 100 000 in the south. In the West, incidence generally is lower, but France and Switzerland have high rates. In the USA, incidence is three times higher in the Black American population than amongst whites. In general, cancer of the oesophagus occurs more often in older people (over 55) and is twice as common in men as in women.

Causes

The wide geographical variations in incidence point strongly to environmental factors, especially poor nutrition, as the most common cause of oesophageal cancer. This is one of the few cancers in which heavy alcohol consumption almost certainly plays a part, and heavy smoking too is implicated. Drinking and smoking together seem to increase the risk further. Rarely, other conditions such as achalasia, the loss of the normal contractions of the oesophagus, and narrowing of the oesophagus, which may happen after an accident involving the swallowing of caustic liquids, may also lead to the development of this cancer.

Presentation

The most common symptom of cancer of the oesophagus is difficulty in swallowing—a feeling that food is getting stuck in the gullet—caused by the tumour constricting the oesophagus. Other common symptoms are weight loss, heartburn, or discomfort behind the breast bone, vomiting the day after eating, and very occasionally vomiting blood.

Anyone who has swallowing difficulties, especially if they are also losing weight, should see their doctor to have these symptoms investigated. Although there are other conditions which might cause these problems, tests to exclude oesophageal cancer should be performed.

Investigations

If the symptoms indicate the possibility of oesophageal cancer, the first test is likely to be a barium swallow. For this, the patient will be asked to drink a liquid containing barium, a substance which shows up on X-ray. The doctor can watch on an X-ray machine as the barium flows down the oesophagus, and can note any narrowing of the oesophagus which might be caused by a tumour.

If this test indicates the possibility of a cancer, an endoscopy (an oesophagoscopy) will be performed. For this test a long flexible tube will be passed down the throat into the oesophagus. The doctor can look through this tube (endoscope) and examine the inside of the oesophagus. Samples of suspicious tissue (a biopsy) can be taken through the endoscope for examination under the microscope.

Sedation is given before an oesophagoscopy in order to produce good relaxation and to reduce any discomfort during the test. An anaesthetic may also be sprayed onto the back of the throat to prevent gagging when the tube is passed down.

If the biopsy shows that cancer is present, further tests will be done to see whether the cancer can be removed by surgery, and to check for any spread of the disease.

Ultrasound imaging is a similar procedure to oesophagoscopy. In this test, a tiny ultrasound probe is attached to the end of the endoscope, which allows the doctor to gain a deeper view of the wall of the oesophagus and the surrounding area. This allows the doctor to judge whether the tumour is operable, and to see whether the local lymph glands have been affected by the cancer.

A CT scan (see p.38) may be used to check whether the tumour is operable and to see whether there is any spread of the disease to other parts of the body.

An ultrasound scan of the abdomen (see p.38) may also be carried out to check for evidence of spread.

Treatment

Surgery

Surgery is the treatment of choice, if the cancer has not spread outside the oesophagus. The most common operation removes the section containing the tumour completely and joins the stomach to the remaining short length of oesophagus. Sometimes it may be necessary to use a piece of bowel to join the oesophagus to the stomach—a colonic interposition.

On recovery from the surgery it should be possible to eat normally, although the stomach may be smaller than before and it may be necessary to eat smaller meals more often than previously, and to eat more slowly. Some people find that they experience acid indigestion, or diarrhoea. These problems are quite common, and it is useful to experiment with different foods to see which foods are the most troublesome. The doctor can also give advice on simple treatment for these symptoms, which is very effective.

Radiotherapy

When the cancer is outside the oesophagus itself, and cannot be operated upon, but has not spread to other parts of the body, radiotherapy alone used to be the standard treatment. This was effective in controlling the cancer for a while, but the cancer tended to return, both locally and elsewhere.

Recently it has been shown that combining chemotherapy with radiotherapy substantially improves the outcome for people in this situation, some of whom achieve long-term cure. Nowadays, chemotherapy combined with radiotherapy is standard treatment, except for people who are too unfit to undergo chemotherapy.

Radiotherapy is also very useful to relieve symptoms caused by narrowing of the oesophagus, as it shrinks the tumour, making swallowing easier and relieving discomfort.

Chemotherapy

Following the markedly improved results shown in people treated with a combination of chemotherapy and radiotherapy, further research is now going on to see if the same combination of treatment can cause tumours which would previously been considered inoperable to shrink sufficiently to become operable. For people with more advanced disease, chemotherapy is often given on its own, and may be very useful in shrinking and controlling the cancer.

Chemotherapy regimens for oesophageal cancer are based on the drug 5-fluorouracil, usually in combination with cisplatinum. Side-effects may include nausea and vomiting and diarrhoea, but these can be well controlled with drugs. This drug combination does not usually cause hair loss.

Relief of symptoms

For people whose cancer cannot be operated on, and who are troubled by problems with swallowing, there are a number of treatments which may be used to alleviate these difficulties.

Intubation is a procedure by which a metal or plastic tube is inserted in the oesophagus to keep it open and to ease swallowing and eating difficulties. Alternatively, the doctor may use a dilator to enlarge the space in the oesophagus. This is a simple and quick procedure but it may need to be repeated after a while.

A bypass operation may be carried out instead of intubation. In this procedure, a piece of the colon is used to create an alternative channel to the stomach, bypassing the tumour obstructing the oesophagus.

Laser therapy may be used to remove enough of the tumour to allow food to pass easily down the oesophagus. Several sessions of treatment may be necessary, and the treatment may need to be repeated to keep the oesophagus clear enough to eat and drink normally.

People who have swallowing difficulties, or who have had a tube fitted will probably need to eat a very soft diet and avoid foods which might cause the tube to become blocked. A hospital dietician will be able to give advice on suitable foods.

Prognosis

If the cancer is confined to the oesophagus, and can be completely removed by surgery, the cure rate for this disease is very high. Significant improvements have been made with the use of combined chemotherapy and radiotherapy in people whose cancer is inoperable, some of whom now achieve long-term cure. The optimal combination of surgery, radiotherapy, and chemotherapy can achieve much better results than were possible even a few years ago.

Stomach cancer

Over the past 60 years there has been a most exciting and encouraging decrease in the incidence of stomach cancer in the western world, and this trend is continuing. In the United States, for example, between 1950 and the 1980s the death rate from stomach cancer decreased by 59 per cent in men and 65 per cent in women. Nevertheless, it remains the sixth most common cancer in both men and women, with more than twice as many men as women being affected, and it is more common in older people.

Causes

There are a number of pieces of evidence which indicate that the main causes of stomach cancer are probably environmental. This theory is strongly supported by studies of migrant populations; populations who have moved from their country of origin to live in another country, over a generation or so, adopt the same risk of stomach cancer as natives of that country. The decrease in incidence of stomach cancer over most

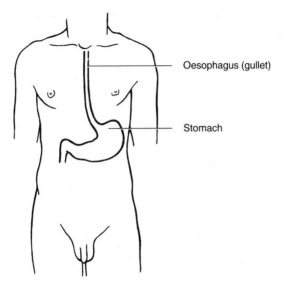

Figure 10 Oesophagus and stomach.

of this century can probably be attributed mainly to the widespread use of refrigeration to preserve food. In parts of the world where traditional methods of food preservation are still common, the incidence of stomach cancer is also much higher—with rates in Japan the highest in the world (78 per 100 000 population as compared to 10 per 100 000 in the USA); eastern Europe and South America also have a very high incidence of the disease.

A diet which includes plenty of fresh vegetables and fruit and is high in fibre may well have a protective effect and reduce the risk of stomach cancer. Smoked, pickled, or salted foods, which are thought to be implicated in its development, should probably be eaten only in moderation.

It is thought that there may be some relationship between the levels of nitrates in drinking water, and incidence of stomach cancer. There does not appear to be any relationship between alcohol consumption and the development of this disease.

People who have a condition called pernicious anaemia, in which the lining of the stomach is thinned and there is a reduction in acid production coupled with a deficiency of the vitamin B12, are known to be at increased risk of developing stomach cancer. There is no proven link, however, between stomach ulcers and the development of stomach cancer.

Presentation

The commonest symptom of stomach cancer is persistent indigestion. Others include discomfort or a bloated feeling in the upper abdomen after eating, possibly associated with nausea and vomiting; loss of appetite; weight loss; occasionally vomiting blood or passing blood in the stools. Many of these symptoms are similar to those of minor, and very common, conditions such as indigestion, and even the more severe are more commonly associated with benign stomach ulcers.

The vague, non-specific nature of these symptoms means that early diagnosis is not easy. As with other cancers, stomach cancer is most likely to be cured if it is detected at an early stage. Unfortunately, however, a tumour may be growing in the stomach for quite some time before it causes any symptoms, and people with those symptoms may initially be treated by their GP for indigestion or stomach ulcers, causing delay before further investigations are made. This means that many stomach cancers are not diagnosed until they are well advanced, when the prospects for cure are not so good.

In Japan, where stomach cancer is very common, anyone with even the most minor symptoms is investigated straight away; most stomach cancers are therefore detected at an early stage, and the long-term survival figures are much better than in the West. Studies in the West have also shown that investigations at the first sign of indigestion would pick up many early stomach cancers. However, this would pose a major problem because indigestion and peptic ulcers are by far the most common explanations for these symptoms, and it is difficult to decide how far everyone with indigestion should be investigated. Certainly, however, anyone over the age of 45 who has persistent indigestion should see their doctor and should be investigated to exclude an ulcer and to make sure there is no evidence of stomach cancer.

Tests

The first test is likely to be a barium meal—a form of X-ray. For this test, the patient is asked to swallow a white liquid containing barium, which shows up on X-ray. The barium outlines the stomach so that it can be seen clearly on an X-ray screen, and the couch on which the patient lies may be tipped in several different positions to allow the barium to flow through the stomach. Any abnormalities of the stomach can be seen on the screen and it is usually possible to see which growths look benign and which are suspicious.

The only way to be certain of a diagnosis is to examine some tissue under the microscope, and so, for a more accurate investigation of any suspicious areas, a gastroscopy will be performed. For this, a long flexible tube will be passed down the patient's throat and gullet (oesophagus) and into the stomach. The doctor can look through this tube and examine the inside of the stomach. Photographs can be taken, and samples of cells taken (a biopsy) through the tube, to be examined under the microscope. For this test, the patient is usually given a sedative, and a local anaesthetic is sprayed onto the back of the throat to prevent discomfort and gagging while the tube is passed down.

If cancer is definitely present, a CT scan (see p.38) will usually be performed to see whether any local lymph glands are involved, whether the liver is affected, and also to enable the surgeon to decide whether or not the tumour can be removed by an operation. An ultrasound scan is another way of looking at the stomach, liver, and lymph glands and may be used instead of a CT scan to give the surgeon similar information.

Treatment

Surgery

Surgery is the commonest and best way of curing stomach cancer. Usually it is possible to remove part of the stomach only (a partial gastrectomy). The local lymph nodes will usually be removed at the same time. If a partial gastrectomy is not possible, a total gastrectomy will be performed, which removes the whole of the stomach, together with a lower part of the gullet and the spleen. In this case, the gullet is reconnected directly to the small intestine.

When people have had part or all of their stomach removed, once they have recovered from the operation, it is generally recommended that they eat several small meals and snacks during the day, rather than few larger meals, as they will probably feel full quite quickly. For this reason, too, it is probably best to take drinks separately from meals. Most people find it takes a bit of time, and trial and error, to find a pattern of eating which suits them, and foods which agree with them. It is very important, however, to try to ensure a good diet, as many people with stomach cancer lose a lot of weight, and need to restore their weight to near normal to aid their recovery. It may be necessary, at least to begin with, to supplement the diet with nutritious drinks, available on prescription or from a chemist. The hospital dietitian should be able to give advice on diet before the patient is discharged.

People who have had gastrectomy operations will probably be deficient in a chemical called intrinsic factor, manufactured in the stomach, which is important for the absorption of vitamin B12. For this reason, supplements of the vitamin will usually be given by injection, at three-monthly intervals, to ensure that people do not suffer a deficiency of this vitamin.

Chemotherapy

Even when the tumour itself and the local lymph glands have been removed surgically, there may be a risk that the cancer has spread to set up tiny metastases, too small to be seen on a scan, which may cause a recurrence of the cancer later on. This is more likely if the lymph nodes are themselves affected by cancer. Studies in Japan have shown that giving chemotherapy to prevent recurrence of the cancer when there is a high risk of relapse (adjuvant chemotherapy) does improve survival rates. Research in the West, however, has not shown the same improvement in survival rates, and therefore the use of adjuvant chemotherapy remains experimental at this time.

Experimental studies are also under way to see whether giving chemotherapy before surgery can shrink the tumour, making it easier to remove with an operation. For people who have advanced disease, which has spread to other parts of the body, chemotherapy can be used to shrink and control the cancer for a period of time, although cure is not currently possible.

Most chemotherapy regimens for gastric cancer are based on the drug 5-fluorouracil (5-FU), usually in combination with other drugs such as cisplatinum or adriamycin. Side-effects may include nausea and vomiting (which can be well controlled with the new generation of anti-sickness drugs), diarrhoea, a sore mouth, and hair loss (if adriamycin is used).

Radiotherapy

Radiotherapy is not commonly used to treat stomach cancer, because other organs near the stomach may be damaged by radiation during treatment. If the cancer is advanced and causing distressing or painful symptoms, radiotherapy may be very effective in relieving these.

Prognosis

If a stomach cancer is diagnosed at an early stage the prospects for cure by surgery are good (more than 50 per cent). However, about 80–90 per cent of cases of stomach cancer are not identified until the cancer is advanced and has spread to the lymph glands and beyond, and in these cases the survival rate after five years is less good.

So although the actual numbers of people affected by this cancer have been and continue to go down, it is clear that research on three fronts is still urgently needed to improve these statistics: better means of diagnosing the disease; more effective adjuvant chemotherapy; and further improvements in controlling the disease and prolonging life.

Rare tumours of the stomach

Leiomyosarcomas

These are cancers of the smooth muscle of the stomach and vary widely in their degree of aggressiveness. They represent less than 1 per cent of all stomach cancers. The majority are treated by surgery to remove the tumour. Chemotherapy is also used, but its role is experimental at the moment.

Non-Hodgkin's lymphomas

These tumours are described on p.38 and respond similarly to treatment. Stomach lymphomas, represent less than 1 per cent of all stomach cancers.

The first line of treatment is usually surgery to remove the stomach, followed by chemotherapy. A rare subtype are known as Mucosal Associated T cell Lymphomas (MALT lymphomas), and these in the early stage may occasionally respond to antibiotics given against infection by a bacterium known as *Helicobacter*.

Bowel cancer

Cancers of the colon and rectum (the large bowel) are the second commonest cancers in men (after lung cancer) and the third commonest in women (after breast and lung cancers), in the western world. These cancers mainly affect people over the age of 40, with approximately similar rates for men and women, although in older age groups, the rates for men are somewhat higher than for women. Cancer of the small bowel is very rare.

Incidence rates in other westernized countries are similar. However, there are very large variations in the incidence of these cancers in different parts of the world, with countries in Asia and Africa having a very much lower incidence; even within Europe there are substantially different rates in different parts of the continent, with countries in northern and western Europe having more cases than countries in the south and east. These facts strongly indicate that cancers of the large bowel are principally diseases of the more affluent western world,

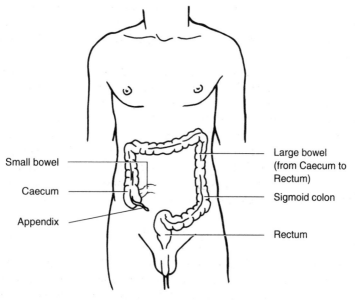

Figure 11   Bowel.

and that environmental factors, especially diet, are probably a major causative factor.

Causes

As mentioned, diet is considered to play an important role in the development of cancers of the colon and rectum, in particularly a high-calorie diet that is rich in meat and animal fats and low in fibre. It has also been suggested that alcohol intake may affect the development of the disease. Conversely, there does seem to be evidence to show that a diet that is rich in fruit and vegetables and fibre and low in fats and alcohol may offer some protection.

Genetic factors play a part in the development of some colorectal cancers. The clearest evidence of this is with people who have a rare inherited condition called familial adenomatous polyposis, in which a number of benign tumours (polyps) develop in the lining of the colon. Anyone with a parent who has this condition has a substantial risk of developing it themselves; and people with the condition have a very high risk of developing cancer of the colon.

Some families seem to have a predisposition to developing cancer of the colon, even though there is no history of familial adenomatous polyposis. If several members of a family have cancer of the colon, especially if it develops at a relatively young age, then the risk that other members of the family might develop the disease is increased.

People who have had inflammatory diseases of the bowel, ulcerative colitis, and, to a lesser extent, Crohn's disease, also have an increased risk of getting bowel cancer.

However, cancers attributable to these risk factors form only a small proportion of the total number of cancers of the bowel that occur; most cases develop spontaneously, and while diet, alcohol consumption, and other environmental factors may be part of the cause, research is still going on to establish clearer links.

Presentation

Cancers of the colon and rectum are nearly 100 per cent curable if picked up in the early stages. It is therefore most important that any symptoms should be checked by a doctor as soon as they are noticed.

The most common symptom of cancer of the large bowel is blood in the stools (faeces). Bleeding after a bowel motion should be investigated. The most likely explanation is of haemorrhoids (piles), but the only way that this can be checked is for the doctor to carry out investigations to exclude bowel cancer. Although these can be a little embarrassing, it is important that these tests are done. If the doctor does not suggest doing any investigations, it is worth asking why not.

A change in bowel habit is another common symptom. If someone has constipation or diarrhoea, or the two conditions alternating, which has lasted for longer than two weeks, then advice should be sought from a doctor. Again, there are many other possible reasons for these symptoms, but they should not be left without being investigated to make sure that there is no underlying bowel cancer at a very early stage, when it is most easily treated.

Pain in the abdomen or back passage are less common symptoms of bowel cancer. Occasionally, if the tumour is causing a blockage or obstruction in the bowel, it might cause symptoms including swelling of the abdomen, cramp-like pains, nausea, vomiting, and constipation. If the disease has spread to other parts of the body, other symptoms might be apparent, such as weight loss and jaundice.

Screening

At the moment there is no general screening programme for bowel cancer. The only practical way to screen large sections of the population is by a faecal occult blood test—testing the stools for minute quantities of blood which are not always apparent to the eye. There are problems with this test, however. It requires people to test their stools on a regular basis and may therefore not be very acceptable to people who are asymptomatic; it yields many false positives, which cause substantial anxiety and have to be followed-up by further tests; and it is quite expensive.

Despite these difficulties, faecal occult blood tests offer the possibility of picking up colon cancer at an early stage when it is most curable. Trials are now in progress to see whether this test does in practice save lives by detecting substantially more cancers at an earlier stage than are found at present, and to see whether it is practical and acceptable to the general population.

For people who have a strong family history of colon cancer, it may be worthwhile considering the benefit of regular screening over the age of 35 or 40, with a faecal occult blood test, and possibly regular colonoscopies also (see below).

Investigations

The first test to establish whether bowel cancer is present is a rectal examination, in which the doctor inserts a gloved finger into the back passage to feel for any lumps or swellings. A sigmoidoscope, a flexible tube, may be inserted into the rectum and up into the lower part of the colon, to allow the doctor to see the lowest 20–25 cm of the bowel, where a very high proportion of tumours occur.

If these tests do not show a clear explanation for the symptoms, the doctor may want to examine the whole length of the large bowel, using an instrument called a colonoscope. For this test, the bowel has to be completely empty, so you, the patient, will be asked to follow a bowel cleansing regime for a day or so before the test, including taking laxatives, drinking plenty of fluids, and having the bowel washed out before the test. The colonoscopy takes place while under sedation, and is not painful, though it can be a bit uncomfortable.

The long flexible tube is passed into the back passage and up into the large bowel. It can pass around the curves of the bowel, and a light enables the doctor to examine the bowel wall for abnormalities. Photographs and biopsies can be taken through the tube for later examination.

An X-ray of the inside of the bowel can be taken using a barium enema (see p.36). Preparation for this test is similar to that for a colonoscopy, as the bowel needs to be completely empty. A mixture of barium and air is passed into the back passage, and a series of X-rays taken. As the barium can be seen on X-ray, the doctor can watch its passage through the bowel on an X-ray screen and will notice any abnormalities or swellings in the bowel wall.

A barium enema is a tiring and rather uncomfortable procedure, and can cause cramping pains. For a couple of days afterwards the stools may be white, as the barium is excreted from the body. A laxative for a few days may be necessary as the barium can cause constipation.

Other tests may be performed to check for spread of the disease to other parts of the body; the most usual are an ultrasound scan (see p.38) of the liver, a CT scan (see p.38.) of the abdomen and liver, and a chest X-ray.

Treatment

Surgery is the main treatment for cancer of the large bowel. The surgeon will aim to remove the tumour itself, with a surrounding margin of healthy tissue. In most cases, the two open ends of the bowel can then be joined together again. During the operation, the adjacent lymph glands will usually be removed as well, as this is the first place to which the disease is likely to spread.

If, for some reason, the two cut ends of bowel cannot be joined together, a colostomy is performed. The open end of the bowel is brought out onto the skin of the abdominal wall, forming a stoma (opening out through the abdominal wall). A bag is worn over the stoma to collect the stool. Sometimes the colostomy is only temporary, and a further operation to rejoin the bowel can be done a few months later. If such an operation is not possible, the colostomy is permanent.

Usually a permanent colostomy is only necessary when the operation site is very low down in the colon, near the rectum, and it is impossible to operate without damaging the function of the anal sphincter which controls the expulsion of the bowel movements.

Advances in surgical techniques have improved many aspects of surgical treatment for people with colon cancer. Fewer people now need to have colostomies. The use of the staple gun, rather than hand sewing, has meant that operations low down in the colon can be done without interfering with the anal sphincter's function. Laparoscopic (keyhole) surgery is a technique in which the surgeon operates through small incisions in the abdomen, rather than by opening up the abdomen completely, allowing patients to recover more quickly. Laparoscopic surgery is still, however, a very new technique and is only performed in a few specialized cancer treatment centres.

Some men who have surgery for cancers very low down in the pelvis may find that the surgery causes damage to the nerves which go to the sexual organs. New nerve-sparing techniques of surgery have been developed to avoid damage wherever possible. If damage does occur, however, a man may not be able to have or maintain an erection, and may have problems with ejaculation. These problems occur very rarely, and may resolve over time but occasionally they are permanent. In such cases, treatment such as injections of papaverine to induce erections, or the implantation of a prosthesis in the penis (which may be semi-rigid, producing a permanently erect penis, or inflatable at will), can be given to minimize the sexual problems caused by cancer surgery.

Living with a colostomy

Although fewer people with cancer of the colon now need to have a colostomy, this is an aspect of bowel cancer treatment which many people dread. Though learning to live with a colostomy is not easy and takes time, many people find that they can get back to all their normal activities after this operation.

In most hospitals there are stoma care nurses, who are specially trained to support and help people who have had colostomies, both in the practical aspects of caring for the stoma and using a colostomy bag, and in the emotional aspects of learning to live with an altered body. Many people, too, find it supportive to talk to people who have had the same operation who can speak from personal experience about ways to cope, and there are support groups specifically for people who have had colostomies.

The surgeon will carefully plan the positioning of the stoma, before the operation, so that the bag stays in place during all normal activities. The stoma care nurse, after the operation, can offer advice on various different kinds of bag and appliance. It may be possible to avoid the necessity of wearing a bag by irrigating, or flushing out the colostomy once a day.

It may be necessary to regulate the diet after a colostomy, as some foods may make the stools loose and cause the colostomy to act too frequently. However, these reactions may settle down after a while. It may be helpful to seek the advice of the hospital dietician if problems continue.

Adjuvant therapy

After the tumour has been removed surgically, it, and any local lymph glands that have been removed, will be examined by a pathologist. The appearance of the tumour under the microscope will suggest how likely it is that the cancer may recur. The most important factors determining this risk are whether the tumour has spread through the bowel wall and, more importantly, whether the local lymph glands have been affected. Even though the tumour and the glands have been completely removed by surgery, if the glands have been affected, it is possible that tiny metastases, too small to be seen on scans, are already established in other parts of the body, and that over time these will grow and cause a recurrence of the cancer.

It is known that chemotherapy is more effective at this stage, when the metastases are extremely small. Therefore, in situations where there is a high risk of relapse, treatment is given to prevent recurrence. This kind of treatment is called adjuvant therapy.

Recent research has shown that adjuvant chemotherapy based on a drug called 5-fluorouracil (5-FU) significantly reduces the risk of relapse and increases the chance of survival. There are a number of different regimens and techniques for giving this drug. Sometimes it is combined with a drug called levamisole, which is thought possibly to increase the body's natural immunity, or with the vitamin folinic acid, which enhances the effectiveness of 5-FU. These drugs are usually given by intravenous injection over a period varying from six months to one year. New research is investigating the effect of giving the drug directly into the vein that supplies blood to the liver.

When the tumour is in the rectum (lower part of the bowel), especially if it has spread through the bowel wall or the lymph glands are involved, there is a high risk that the cancer may return in the pelvis, as well as elsewhere in the body. In this case, adjuvant radiotherapy (radiotherapy given after the operation even when there is no apparent residual disease) to the pelvic area is given, in addition to adjuvant chemotherapy.

Recurrence

If the cancer returns, or has already spread to other parts of the body when first diagnosed, it is usually treated with chemotherapy rather than surgery. The drugs used to treat advanced disease are also based on 5-fluorouracil, usually combined with folinic acid. The aim of treatment is to shrink and control the cancer for as long as possible.

The side-effects of this drug are quite mild; the main ones are a sore mouth, diarrhoea, occasionally nausea. These can usually be well controlled with drugs, and may be prevented completely. Occasionally hair loss may occur; the hair will always grow back again after treatment has finished.

Research continues to investigate the most effective way of giving 5-FU and to look at other drugs which might be given in combination with 5-FU to increase its activity.

If the cancer has come back only in the pelvis, radiotherapy may be given as well, to shrink and control the tumour. Side-effects of radiotherapy may occur for a few weeks after treatment and include nausea, diarrhoea, frequency of urination, and a burning sensation during urination.

If the cancer has come back in a very small area only, for example as a single lesion in one lung, or in one lobe of the liver, an operation to remove the affected part surgically may sometimes be considered if the patient is young and fit.

Prognosis

As mentioned before, cancer of the large bowel has a very high chance of cure if diagnosed at an early stage. However, nearly half of all patients are not diagnosed until their cancer is at a more advanced stage. Overall about half of all patients are cured with surgery combined with adjuvant chemotherapy and radiotherapy, and these cure rates are improving. Undoubtedly, however, the most effective way to improve the rates is by early diagnosis.

For people with a tumour that is still contained within the wall of the bowel, the cure rate is in excess of 80 per cent. If the tumour has spread through the wall, but nowhere else, and no lymph glands are affected, the cure rate is around 70 per cent. If the disease has spread to involve the local lymph glands, the cure rate is between 30 and 50 per cent. These are the people for whom the outcome is likely to be substantially improved with adjuvant treatment.

In people with advanced disease chemotherapy is given with the intention of shrinking the cancer in order to relieve symptoms, improving the quality of life, and of prolonging survival where this is possible.

These statistics indicate the importance of health education to promote awareness of the symptoms of bowel cancer, to stress the importance of vigilance about symptoms, and to overcome the hesitation and embarrassment people may have in talking about such symptoms to their doctor and having them investigated.

Rare tumours of the bowel

Cancer of the small bowel

These are very rare tumours (usually adenocarcinomas) which occur most commonly in the duodenum. They often cause blockage of the small bowel, and symptoms of the blockage are likely to be the first sign of their presence. They are usually treated by surgery, although some experimental treatment with chemotherapy has shown good results.

Lymphomas of the small bowel

These cancers also present with symptoms of bowel obstruction, including nausea and vomiting, possibly diarrhoea. They are more common in people who have Crohn's disease (an inflammatory condition of the bowel). The standard treatment is surgery to remove the tumour, followed by chemotherapy, with good results.

Carcinoid tumours

These most commonly occur in the appendix and the small bowel, although they may occur in the lung or pancreas or, rarely, in any other part of the body. When a carcinoid tumour lies in the appendix it often causes very few problems and is very unlikely to spread (90 per cent never metastasize). Many such tumours are only discovered because investigations for some other problem show them up.

Carcinoids outside the appendix do metastasize, especially to the liver. They secrete a chemical called serotonin which can cause flushing and diarrhoea. The symptoms can be controlled effectively with a newly available drug, somatostatin.

Initial treatment, if there are no metastases, is to remove the primary tumour by surgery. A significant proportion of tumours respond to chemotherapy based on 5-fluorouracil which can shrink and control the tumour but not cure it. Interferon can also be helpful in controlling the cancer.

Cancer of the pancreas

Cancer of the pancreas is the sixth commonest cancer and the fourth most common cause of cancer deaths in adults. It occurs predominantly in older age groups, and is slightly more common in men than in women.

There has been an increase in incidence of this cancer (as much as five-fold in some regions) in the western world throughout the twentieth century, though there are very wide variations between countries. Studies of immigrant populations in the USA have shown that among first generation immigrants the incidence of pancreatic cancer is the same as in their country of origin, but among subsequent generations, the incidence tends to follow the same pattern as that of the white American population. Environmental causes therefore seem very likely to be significant factors in the development of this cancer, but no definite associations have been made. There seems to be a very slightly increased risk among cigarette smokers, although this is by no means as clear cut as the link between smoking and lung cancer. There seems also to be a slightly increased risk for people affected by chronic pancreatitis.

Presentation

As with other cancers of the gastro-intestinal system, pancreatic cancer often presents with very vague and non-specific symptoms. The most common is pain in the upper abdomen and back, possibly associated with a poor appetite and weight loss. If the tumour has developed in the head of the pancreas through which the bile duct passes, it may block the bile duct, preventing bile from being carried from the liver to the intestine. This blockage results in components of the bile accumulating in the blood, causing jaundice (yellowing of the skin and the whites of the eyes, while the urine becomes dark yellow and the stools become pale). This is not usually associated with pain.

These symptoms may be caused by many conditions other than pancreatic cancer, but a doctor should be consulted if jaundice or any persistent abdominal symptoms develop so that they can be investigated.

Investigations

The doctor may be able to feel a lump in the pancreas by gently feeling the abdomen. A barium meal is usually required at an early stage of the investigations, to find out whether the symptoms are caused by some other cause such as stomach ulcers. This test is described on p. 36. The barium coats the stomach and intestine so that the outlines can be seen clearly on an X-ray screen, and any narrowing of these organs caused by a swelling in the pancreas pressing on them can also be seen.

If the physical examination, and/or the barium meal have not definitely excluded pancreatic cancer, the next test is likely to be an ultrasound scan (see p.38) of the abdomen followed by an ERCP (see below) then, a CT scan (see p. 38). These will give a picture of the pancreas, showing any lump as well as the local lymph glands and the liver, so that the doctor can see whether there has been any spread of the disease. It is often possible for the doctor to take a small sample of cells (a biopsy) for examination under a microscope, during the CT scan. A local anaesthetic is used to numb the area and the doctor can then insert a needle into any suspicious mass, guided by the picture on the CT scan.

Occasionally, even after all these tests, there is still no firm diagnosis. In this case, an operation called a laparotomy may be performed under a general anaesthetic to remove a small piece of tissue from the pancreas. This is usually only done if surgery is being considered as treatment, as the tissue can be examined immediately, and the surgeon can proceed to do a further operation straight away if the diagnosis is confirmed.

Treatment

Surgery

Surgery is only possible in a minority of people. The intention is to remove the entire tumour if the cancer has not spread beyond the pancreas, and the patient is fairly young and otherwise fit. Depending on where the cancer is situated, it may be necessary to remove part or all of the pancreas. It may also be necessary to remove a part of the stomach and the duodenum, the common bile duct and the surrounding glands at the same time.

After such an operation, it will be necessary to take capsules of pancreatic enzymes and to have injections of insulin to replace the substances normally provided by the pancreas. If the tumour cannot be removed and it is obstructing the bile duct, causing jaundice, various surgical procedures can be used to relieve the blockage.

An ERCP (Endoscopic Retrograde Cholangio Pancreatography – involves placing a catheter in the biliary tree and injecting a radio-opaque dye), allows the doctor to see the narrowed part of

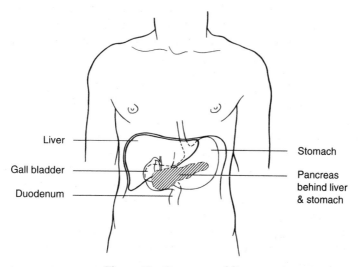

Figure 12 Pancreas and liver.

the bile duct on the X-ray screen. He or she can insert dilators into the narrowing to stretch it, then insert a plastic tube, about 5 to 10 cm long, through the endoscope. The bile can then drain properly again, and symptoms caused by the build-up of bile products, such as jaundice, will quickly go. The tube will probably have to be replaced every three to four months to prevent it becoming blocked, but very few people suffer any side-effects from ERCP.

A similar procedure called percutaneous transhepatic cholangiography (PTC) can also be used to position a stent to drain a blocked bile duct. In the same way, a dye is used to show up the blockage or narrowing on an X-ray screen. After a local anaesthetic has numbed the abdominal area, a needle is inserted through the skin just below the rib cage. A guide wire is passed through the needle, then through the blockage in the bile duct and out into the duodenum. A plastic stent can then be passed along this guide wire and placed in position. This procedure will probably require a few days' stay in hospital, and antibiotics to prevent any infection.

If neither of these methods is possible, operations to bypass the blockage may be suggested. The most common way is to join the gall bladder to part of the bowel (the jejunum), allowing the bile to flow directly from the liver to the intestine. This operation is called a cholecystojejunostomy.

If the duodenum (the first part of the intestine) is blocked by pressure from the tumour in the pancreas, causing persistent vomiting, an operation can be performed to bypass the duodenum by connecting a piece of the bowel (the jejunum) to the stomach.

Radiotherapy

Radiotherapy may be given to people who have had surgery to remove a tumour in the pancreas, in order to control any tiny foci of cancer that may have been left behind. More recently, doctors have begun to investigate the use of radiotherapy before surgery, to shrink the tumour and to improve the chances that the whole tumour can be removed. With this, some tumours which would previously have been considered inoperable can now be treated surgically. Other recent research has shown that radiotherapy combined with chemotherapy (see below) may give improved results on cancers that are not operable but have not spread beyond the pancreas. Radiotherapy can be very helpful also in controlling pain in people whose cancer cannot be operated upon.

The side-effects of radiotherapy to the abdomen can be unpleasant and can include nausea, vomiting and diarrhoea, but usually these can be well controlled with drugs, and they resolve after the course of treatment has ended.

Chemotherapy

Chemotherapy has a limited role in the treatment of cancer of the pancreas and its use is still under evaluation. As mentioned above, some improvement has been shown when chemotherapy is used together with radiotherapy, for inoperable tumours that have not spread. Drug regimens are based on the drug 5-fluorouracil (5FU), and common side-effects include nausea and vomiting, diarrhoea and a sore mouth, which can be prevented or well controlled with drugs.

Hormonal treatment

Many pancreatic tumours have high levels of oestrogen receptors in the cells—proteins which take up oestrogen from the blood and encourage the cell to grow. There is now some evidence to show that tamoxifen (see p. 97), a drug which prevents the receptors in the cancer cells from taking up oestrogen, may be helpful in prolonging survival.

Pain relief

Persistent pain can be a distressing problem for people with cancer of the pancreas. Injections of chemicals to numb the nerves to the pancreas can be given from the onset of the pain, and can be very helpful in relieving it.

Prognosis

Surgical removal of the tumour leads to cure in a few people with cancer of the pancreas. In others, however, the disease returns because of microscopic disease which cannot be removed at operation. For people whose cancer cannot be removed, treatment is given with the aim of controlling symptoms and giving a good quality of life. Cure is not possible with current modalities of treatment.

Research in this field is concentrating on the use of radiotherapy and chemotherapy as treatment for inoperable cancers and for their use both before and after an operation to improve the results of surgical treatment.

Rare tumours of the pancreas

Carcinoid tumours

These can occur as primary tumours of the pancreas. When they do, they behave very similarly to the more common carcinoid tumours of the gastro-intestinal tract, see p.134.

Neuroendocrine tumours and islet cell tumours

A number of uncommon tumours of the pancreas produce hormones. These include carcinoid tumours (which produce a chemical called 5HIAA), islet cell tumours (which produce insulin), and others which produce hormones which act on the gastro-intestinal tract. Some tumours do not secrete hormones and these are described as non-functional. If such tumours are diagnosed in the early stages, while they are small, they can be removed surgically. Alternatively they may respond to radiotherapy. For tumours which cannot be cured, interferon may have a role in shrinking and controlling the cancer, and chemotherapy with 5-fluorouracil or a drug known as streptozocin have some activity against the tumour.

Cancer of the liver

The liver is one of the commonest sites to which cancers in other parts of the body may spread, and most cancers found in the liver are secondaries and not primary liver cancer. Many cancers have the potential to spread to the liver, and liver metastases are therefore fairly common. Primary liver cancer is however uncommon in the western world, but occurs quite frequently in Africa and some parts of Asia. This chapter mainly discusses primary liver cancer.

There are two main kinds of liver cancer; those which arise in the cells of the liver itself, which are called hepatomas, and those which arise in the bile ducts, which are called cholangiocarcinomas if they arise within the liver, and bile duct carcinomas if they arise in the part of the duct which is outside the liver. Bile duct cancers are much less common than hepatomas.

In developed countries, primary liver cancer is a disease of middle-aged and elderly people and occurs twice as often in men than in women. Most of these people who develop hepatoma usually already have cirrhosis of the liver—scarring of the liver caused by heavy alcohol drinking over many years. Occasionally hepatomas arise as a complication of hepatitis which has become chronic. Both these conditions are relatively common, but cancer of the liver is an uncommon complication.

In rare instances, a condition called haemachromatosis, which causes increased deposits of iron throughout the body including the liver, may lead to the development of a hepatoma.

In Africa and Asia, primary cancer of the liver is very much more common and occurs in young people in their 20s and 30s, whose livers are not damaged by alcohol. It is thought that exposure to aflatoxins—fungi found in grains and beer—may be the cause. There is also a strong association with hepatitis. Infection with a parasite called the liver fluke is thought possibly to be a cause for many bile duct cancers.

Presentation

The symptoms of both primary and secondary liver cancers are similar. Often the first sign is discomfort and perhaps swelling in the upper abdomen, caused by enlargement of the liver. People may feel generally unwell—tired, with loss of appetite, nausea and weight loss, and sometimes a high temperature with shivery, flu-like symptoms.

If the cancer is blocking the bile duct, preventing the passage of bile from the liver to the intestine, products from the bile may build up in the blood causing jaundice. This makes the skin and whites of the eyes go yellow, and the skin may become itchy. The urine becomes very dark in colour and the faeces become a pale chalky colour.

Sometimes fluid called ascites may build up in the abdomen causing it to swell. There are a number of reasons why this build-up of fluid may occur: it may be that cancer cells from the liver have spread to the lining of the abdomen and irritate it; it may be that damage to the liver upsets the normal balance of fluid in the body; or it may be that cancer cells are causing a blockage in the venous drainage from the abdomen, preventing the normal drainage of fluid.

Jaundice, and build-up of fluid in the abdomen, may be caused by many other conditions than liver cancer. However, they do always indicate a condition that needs medical attention, and if they develop medical advice should be sought without delay.

Tests

A physical examination of the abdomen is the first test that a doctor will carry out. It is often possible for the doctor to feel if the liver is enlarged; it may be quite hard and will feel tender. An ultrasound or CT scan (see p.38) of the liver will usually enable the doctor to see whether there is a tumour in the liver, and to check its extent. If the doctor suspects primary liver cancer, the next test is likely to be a blood test to check the levels of a chemical called alpha-fetoprotein. Raised levels of this substance would indicate the likely diagnosis of a hepatoma.

If the doctor knows that a primary cancer already exists in another part of the body, there is probably no need to take a sample of cells from the tumour in the liver for examination under the microscope. However, if there is no known primary cancer, then a biopsy will be necessary to make a definite diagnosis. The biopsy is done under local anaesthetic, but will probably entail an overnight stay in hospital. The doctor will use ultrasound or CT scanning to locate the tumour exactly, then remove a small sample using a needle. If the results of this test show that the liver cancer is a secondary, further tests will be done to locate the primary from which it stems. If the results of the biopsy show primary liver cancer there will probably be no need for further tests, as this kind of cancer seldom spreads outside the abdomen.

Treatment

Surgery

If only one part of the liver is affected by the cancer and the rest of the liver functions satisfactorily and has not been severely damaged by cirrhosis, it may be possible to remove the affected part. The liver has an amazing capacity to repair itself, and will start to regrow even if half or three-quarters of it has been removed. Sadly, however, in many people the tumour is too large, or there are a number of tumours in the liver, and surgical removal is not possible.

Liver transplantation may also be considered in primary cancer of the liver. Unfortunately, in the majority of people the cancer recurs in the transplanted liver. However, some people may live for a long time following transplantation especially when the tumours in the excised liver were small.

This procedure is still experimental and its role should become clear in the next few years.

Surgery does not usually play a role in the treatment of secondary liver cancer. Very occasionally, however, if there are only one or two foci of cancer in the liver, and very careful screening has shown no other secondaries anywhere else in the body, an operation to remove the affected parts of the liver may be done.

Chemotherapy

Chemotherapy's role in treating primary liver cancer is not yet proven, but many studies are going on to investigate ways of improving outcome. Drugs have been used successfully to shrink and control liver cancer for a while, in some people.

For secondary liver cancer, the success of chemotherapy depends on the sensitivity of the primary cancer to certain drugs. If a primary cancer is very chemosensitive, then the liver metastases will be too.

An experimental method of delivering chemotherapy drugs is to put them directly into the artery that supplies the blood to the liver. In this way, larger doses of drugs can be given directly to the tumour with fewer side-effects on the rest of the body.

Radiotherapy

The liver is extremely sensitive to radiation and is easily damaged with quite small doses, so this form of treatment is not often used.

Laser therapy and alcohol injections

If a few small secondary tumours remain after chemotherapy, doctors are experimenting with two new treatments to try to eliminate them. One is by burning out the remaining lesions with a laser beam. The other is to destroy the tumour by injecting alcohol directly into it. These methods are still under evaluation.

Prognosis

Primary liver cancer is difficult to treat. A minority of people with this cancer are cured by surgical removal of the affected part of the liver, but for most people, the aim of treatment is to control the cancer and to relieve symptoms.

The results of treating secondary cancer of the liver depend on the source of the primary cancer. With some of the most chemosensitive kinds of primary cancer (for example teratomas, see p. 155–160) it is possible to cure people even if they have metastases in the liver. But again, for most people with liver metastases, the aim of treatment is to control the cancer and provide a good quality of life.

Cancer of the adrenal gland

There are two adrenal glands, one on the upper pole of each kidney. These are very specialized glands which release their secretions (which are concerned with the maintenance of blood pressure and the response to stress) directly into the blood.

Cancers of these glands are very rare. Tumours of the outer area of the gland are often benign (that is they do not have the characteristics of cancer) but since they overproduce the hormones secreted by the normal gland they can cause various changes generally. Those of the outer part of the adrenal gland are called 'adrenocortical tumours' which may be associated with 'Cushing's Syndrome' (see below). Two main types of tumour develop from the core (the medulla) of the adrenal: neuroblastoma—this is essentially a cancer of childhood (see p.195–197); phaeochromocytoma—only about 10 per cent of these are true cancers.

Presentation

The best recognized of these is 'Cushing's syndrome' in which several changes occur: fat develops on the trunk particularly over the back on the shoulders, while the muscles of the upper arms and legs become wasted, the skin thins. In women there may be a male growth of hair on the face and body. Diabetes may also develop. These symptoms may also be caused by a cancer of the adrenal gland and whether benign or not the best treatment is clearly to remove the tumour.

Phaeochromocytomas produce the substances which influence blood pressure and our response to stress so that they may produce a wide range of symptoms such as sudden onset of sweating, faintness, chest discomfort, palpitations, headaches, mood changes, excessive thirst, and large volumes of urine. These tumours are more common in middle age.

Investigation

The clinical picture will already have given the doctor a strong indication of whether the problem is more likely to lie in the cortex or the medulla of the adrenal. This will influence the choice of tests, for example if a tumour of the cortex is suspected then it will be necessary to measure the level in the blood of the hormone produced by the pituitary gland in the brain which drives the adrenal gland (a high level would suggest that the problem is in the pituitary and not in the adrenal); whatever the tumour type a CT scan may show which gland is enlarged—this will probably include the abdomen to check that there has been no spread to the lungs or the liver. A radioisotope scan of the bones can be helpful if there is any suggestion that the cancer is more widespread. Sometimes the cancer does not produce any hormones in which case it is more likely to be discovered when it is large enough to produce symptoms in the abdomen (discomfort, a feeling of fullness, backache, and even a swelling which can be felt in the abdomen). This is unusual in the case of phaeochromocytoma but may occur in very rare cases of tumours arising in the outer rim of the adrenal.

Treatment

Surgical removal is possible in most people, and although the gland is small it is fairly inaccessible so be prepared for a larger scar than seems necessary. In the case of phaeochromocytoma the effects of the hormones produced by the tumour have to be very closely monitored before and during the operation and then the blood pressure controlled during the period of stabilization once the tumour has been removed—giving additional fluids into a vein may be all that is needed. As mentioned in Chapter 6 (p.41) meta-iodobenzyguanidine (MIBG) is taken up by phaeochromocytomas and this can be coupled with a radioactive isotope. If this is injected into a vein the isotope is taken into the tumour and may kill sufficient of the cells to produce relief of symptoms and even a reduction in the size of metastases.

In the very rare situations where cancers of the cortex have spread to distant sites chemotherapy using a drug called mitotane (o,p-DDD, which is related to DDT!) can produce temporary benefit in about a quarter of people who are treated. The side-effects of mitotane are loss of appetite, nausea, sickness, and sometimes diarrhoea. Lethargy and sleepiness are also common while skin changes and vertigo are less so. Chemotherapy may occasionally produce responses.

Urological cancers

The urological system includes all those organs and structures which are involved in the filtration of the blood to produce urine and then its collection and excretion. The principal organs are the kidneys and the bladder—the kidney drains urine to the bladder via drainage tubes called ureters and the bladder drains to the outside via another tube called the urethra. In men the prostate lies at the base of the bladder (the urethra passes through it) and so is included in this section along with the testes and the penis. Cancers can occur in any of these structures (see individual cancers). Those involving the ureters and the urethra are very rare.

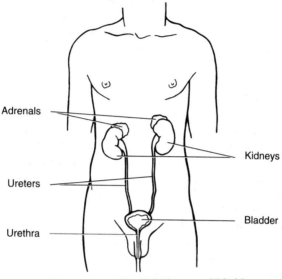

Figure 13   Adrenal, kidney, and bladder.

Cancers of the kidney

Cancers of the kidney are very rare, and in the huge population of the USA only about 8000 people die of cancers of the kidney each year. This is twice the number diagnosed each year in the UK. Most of these are found in adults and are commoner from the sixth decade onwards. They are of the type called 'renal cell carcinoma' or 'hypernephroma'. There is some evidence that cigarette smoking may in some way play a role in the development of this cancer which is three times more common in men than women. One of the commonest tumours in childhood (but even so, extremely rare) also arises in the kidney; this is a 'nephroblastoma' otherwise known as 'Wilm's tumour' (see p.197–198).

Presentation

Renal cell cancer may make itself known in many different ways. As it grows it may cause leakage of blood in the urine. Often the amount is small and this may be missed unless there is a reason for a simple dipstick test to be carried out on the urine. This can be positive for blood even when the amounts are so small that it can only be seen when the urine is examined under a microscope. The growth of the cancer in the kidney may be felt as a lump within the abdomen and this may or may not be associated with discomfort in the loin on the side of the affected kidney. These are the commonest ways in which the cancer makes itself known. Less commonly, some people experience fevers or symptoms caused by the spread (metastasis) of the cancer. In the lungs this may cause shortness of breath and/or cough—occasionally of blood-stained spit; in bone it may cause pain or weakness which can cause a fracture. It is important to tell the doctor about the symptoms being experienced for none of these on their own is enough to prove that a cancer of the kidney exists and he will have to decide which tests are most likely to be helpful.

Investigation

Apart from some routine blood tests which check the blood components, kidney and liver function, a urine test for blood, and a routine chest X-ray, the most useful tests include an IVP (see p.38) an ultrasound examination of the abdomen, or a CT scan of the chest and abdomen (see p.38). An advantage of the CT scan is that the precise localization of any abnormality can be seen in three dimensions and the doctor may be able, using a special needle and a local anaesthetic, to take a biopsy which can be used to make a precise diagnosis without the need for an operation to do this. If the tests show that renal cell cancer is present a bone scan (p.41) may be carried out to see whether there is any sign that the cancer has spread to a bone.

Treatment

If there is no evidence from these tests that the cancer has spread beyond the kidney then an operation will be advised. Most surgeons aim to remove the entire affected kidney, even so it is not always possible to remove the tumour completely. The pathologist is able to give some idea (but it is only an idea) of how completely the tumour has been removed. Even if the surrounding structures which looked suspicious to the surgeon are completely cut out at the operation there can be no certainty that a few cancer cells do not remain. The best test of success is that with the passage of time the cancer does not come back. Even when it is not possible to remove the tumour completely the operation may significantly reduce some of the symptoms such as local discomfort and bleeding into the urine. Post-operative radiotherapy is not routinely given since the area which needs to be treated is fairly large and side-effects such as nausea, diarrhoea, and a fall in blood counts can be troublesome. The side-effects are less of a concern if treatment needs to be given to a bone and as higher doses can be given to a small area, radiotherapy can be quite useful in reducing discomfort and promoting healing.

If the tests have shown only a solitary metastasis then provided the main tumour can be removed, and depending on the site, surgery to remove this together with the kidney may be considered.

When the disease is more widespread and surgery is not possible then the strategy of treatment is to control symptoms. Long tried hormone treatment with medroxyprogesterone acetate is given with the intention of controlling and if possible shrinking the tumour. Useful responses can be obtained in a few people with newer treatments including drugs such as alpha-interferon and an improvement in quality of life is a real prospect. Chemotherapy is not usually effective but new drugs are being tried.

Outlook

This is significantly related to the extent of the cancer at the time of presentation to the doctor. If the cancer is found to be confined within the kidney with no evidence of spread through the outer capsule then two thirds of people are alive and well five years later. This figure diminishes if there is local spread but a significant proportion are still cured.

A rare cancer of the kidney (less than 10 per cent of kidney cancers) *cancer of the renal pelvis* starts in the drainage system of the kidney. The symptoms may be similar to those described above, namely blood in the urine and local discomfort. These cancers look the same under the microscope as the cancers which arise in the bladder, as do those which start lower down in the ureter (the tube draining from the kidney to the bladder). *Cancer of the ureter* may present with pain on passing urine which does not respond to antibiotics and the need to pass urine frequently. The treatment for cancers of the renal pelvis and for those of the ureter is surgery, which may also involve removing part of the bladder—drug treatments similar to those used for bladder cancer may also be used.

Cancer of the bladder

This is one of the first cancers for which a cause was identified. In the 1800s it was noted that workers in the dye industry had a higher incidence of bladder cancer than found generally. This was later found to be due to a cancer promoting substance (a carcinogen) betanaphthylamine. A higher incidence has also been found in workers in the rubber industry, in smokers, and in those infected by a tropical parasite which burrows into the bladder wall. This particular form of 'schistosomiasis', as it is called, is a cause of the high incidence of bladder cancer found in parts of Egypt. In the UK about 13 000 new cases of bladder cancer are diagnosed each year, of these two thirds are in men—the higher incidence being attributed to smoking habits.

Presentation

Blood in the urine may be caused by a variety of problems, not all of them malignant, but it should always be investigated. It is one of the commonest presenting features of bladder cancer. Other symptoms which may occur are an urgent feeling of needing to pass urine, increased frequency of passing water (including during the night), or occasionally a poor stream. If the drainage from the kidney is blocked the back-pressure may cause back pain.

Investigation

Cystoscopy (see p.42) is the most important of the investigations used to make a diagnosis as this allows a direct visual assessment of the tumour (or tumours, as they may be multiple) and their size and location. Biopsies can be taken from suspicious areas. As this is usually performed under general anaesthetic the surgeon can also feel the bladder area through the relaxed muscles of the abdomen and through the rectum.

An IVP is carried out to assess the drainage system as a whole and a

CT scan to provide additional information about the bladder wall and the relationship of any tumour to related structures. A more extensive CT scan may be carried out if there is any suggestion of spread to distant sites such as the lungs or the liver. A bone scan is useful if bone metastases are suspected.

Treatment

The management of bladder cancers is determined by their extent. A complicated system is used for recording this in a series of groupings called stages. A distinction is drawn between those cancers which are limited to the lining membrane of the bladder 'superficial tumours'—these may be single or multiple but once cancer cells have been found the whole membrane is regarded as unstable and at risk of developing new cancers and so must be watched at regular intervals. Regular cystoscopy is advised for anyone who has a superficial bladder cancer with local treatment through the cystoscope for small fronds or nodules using diathermy (heat), cryotherapy (cold), or laser (intense light generating heat). Anti-cancer drugs instilled into the bladder are being assessed in early (superficial) bladder cancer as this form of treatment may have a role in preventing or delaying recurrence. Although it is regarded as 'early' it is taken seriously since in about 10 per cent of people more extensive disease develops needing more substantial treatment.

The next grouping is of 'invasive' cancer. Here the decision on the type of surgery depends on whether fairly straightforward surgical excision is possible or whether some form of reconstruction is neccessary. In the latter case, as for example when the whole bladder has to be removed, a new drain is fashioned from a piece of bowel (a urostomy) and this drains out through the wall of the abdomen. This procedure although valuable in terms of cancer treatment requires a period of adjustment—common problems are of learning to use a urostomy and overcoming feelings of sexual unattractiveness.

The choice of treatment will depend on the size and site of the cancer and so may involve radiotherapy alone, radiotherapy followed by surgery, or surgery alone. Radiotherapy alone may have a place in people with more advanced tumours who might otherwise require an ileal conduit. Chemotherapy prior to surgery (neo adjuvant chemotherapy) is increasingly being used and this may make some inoperable tumours resectable.

Where the cancer recurs, in people with very advanced disease or in those who have distant metastases at presentation, chemotherapy is usually considered. A proportion of people treated experience some shrinkage of the tumour which may be significant enough to produce a valuable improvement in quality of life with a reduction in pain and control of blood loss in the urine. The side-effects of chemotherapy may be worse in those in poor condition and may be difficult to give if the kidney function is poor. The main intention of treatment with chemotherapy is to try to reduce the growth of the cancer and so to improve the quality of life. If radiotherapy has been given previously it will not be possible to repeat this, however, if not it can be very helpful in controlling symptoms.

Prognosis

For superficial tumours three quarters of patents are alive and well at five years and for invasive cancers more than a third will achieve long-term survival. Once the disease is more extensive long-term survival falls substantially.

Living with a urostomy

It takes some time to get used to living with a urostomy but with time most people find it becomes routine and does not interfere with their daily lives. Modern bags are flat and odour free and cannot be noticed in normal clothing. The bags are drainable and usually only need to be changed every few days. A normal diet and fluid intake (including alcohol) are usually not a problem but obviously a larger fluid intake means that the bag will have to be changed more often. Most sports are possible although contact sports are better avoided.

Cancer of the prostate

This cancer has an incidence which increases sharply with age from the sixth decade onwards (95 per cent of prostate cancers occur between the ages of 45 and 80). Since the expectation of life has substantially increased, cancer of the prostate is now one of the commonest cancers in men. No obvious cause is known but there are striking differences in incidence around the world—for example in the USA the incidence and death rate from prostate cancer in black men is almost twice as high as in white men.

Presentation

Early prostate cancer does not usually produce symptoms, only when the collection of cells is large enough to cause pressure on the urethra (the tube leading from the base of the bladder through the prostate and along the penis) are symptoms likely to occur and these are identical to the symptoms produced by benign enlargement of the prostate. The symptoms can include: difficulty or frequency and/or pain on passing water; having to get up often at night to pass water. It is unusual to find blood in the urine.

A common site to which prostate cancer spreads is the bones of the lower back—when this happens it frequently causes backache. It should be remembered that backache is common with increasing age and so this is not necessarily sinister.

Investigation

The doctor will need to carry out an examination of the prostate by inserting a gloved finger into the rectum. This allows him to feel the prostate—by doing so he can gain the impression of whether it is enlarged and whether there is any suggestion of a nodule. Blood tests which are sometimes helpful in indicating a high likelihood of prostate cancer will be arranged. Unfortunately normal blood tests do not exclude cancer and so if cancer is suspected a biopsy will be needed. This can usually be carried out during a rectal examination in out-patients using a special biopsy needle. This is a painless procedure but may occasionally be followed by a brief period during which blood may be passed in the urine.

Prostate cancer can also be a chance finding when it is diagnosed after examining the bits of prostate removed during a 'transurethral resection of the prostate' (TUR)—that is removal of most of the prostate via the urethra. This is carried out in someone whose prostate is enlarged but thought to be non-cancerous.

There is a special blood test for cancer of the prostate (called PSA) but as it is not always abnormal it can only be used for monitoring treatment in those whose levels are abnormal before any treatment is started (including surgery). Other tests which are likely to be arranged are: an isotope bone scan—this is to check whether or not there is spread to any of the bones; an IVP to view the kidneys and the drainage system, within the bladder it may be possible to see irregularities of the prostate; a CT scan of the pelvis—this may be helpful in demonstrating extension of the tumour beyond the capsule of the prostate.

Treatment

Let us first consider those tumours which are either contained within the prostate or have spread only locally. The complications and consequences of extensive surgery (these include loss of sphincter control and impotence) are considerable even in the best hands and have tended to discourage its use in some countries. It is worth remembering that the growth rate of these cancers is often very slow and that it may take ten years for the cancer to become apparent. In older men the slow growth may make treatment less urgent. Radiotherapy is generally more widely used than surgery. Where radiotherapy is possible because the tumour is sufficiently localized the aim is to treat thoroughly—this means that planning of treatment will be quite detailed and may take some time. The radiotherapy beam may be pointed from several different directions in order to get maximum benefit without too much in the way of unpleasant side-effects. Short-term side-effects include diarrhoea, pain on passing urine, and the need to pass urine frequently. While the pain usually clears up within a few weeks the inability to hold water for a long time often remains as the bladder is less able to stretch after high dose radiotherapy.

Where the cancer has spread more widely some form of more general treatment needs to be considered. Since the cancer cells flourish in the presence of male hormones changing these levels or the conditions surrounding the cancer may cause it to shrink. The aim of treatment is to reduce the levels of male hormones which stimulate the growth of the cancer. Castration (the removal of both testicles) has been used as a treatment for about 50 years. It can be very effective in reducing bone pain caused by metastases. An inevitable consequence of removing the major source of male sex hormones is impotence and a profound feeling of loss of masculinity. Newer treatments are now available but castration may still be considered in patients who do not

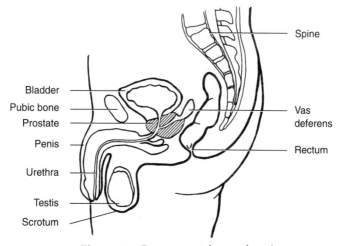

Figure 14   Prostate, urethra, and penis.

want regular follow-up and in those whose severe bone pain is not adequately controlled by other means.

Various hormone treatments are now the treatments of first choice. In the past oestrogen (a female sex hormone) was used and can be very effective but its use is associated with an increased incidence of heart attacks and strokes and also unsightly swelling of the breasts. Newer drugs either work against the male sex hormone or block its release at source (LHRH antagonists). These drugs have fewer side-effects and are now widely used. Recent studies have suggested that combining LHRH antagonists with drugs which block male hormones may increase the effectiveness of treatment.

Chemotherapy has been tried but prostate cancer is not particularly sensitive to the drugs currently available although they may be tried in an attempt to reduce symptoms. Of these the most important is bone pain—if this persists despite hormone therapy then local radiotherapy may be effective in reducing the pain. Alternatively an injection of a radioactive isotope (strontium) into a vein may be helpful as this localizes in the bone metastasis and damages the growing cells.

The careful planning of treatments can make a substantial impact on the quality of life by controlling symptoms even when the disease is widespread.

Prognosis

If the tumour is confined within the capsule of the prostate the five year survival with radiotherapy is very good. Even when it has spread locally long-term control is often possible. Modern treatments now mean that the control of symptoms may be possible for several years.

Cancer of the urethra

These cancers which are exceptionally rare (but more common in women than men), start in the tube draining from the bladder to the outside. They may cause pain on passing urine, or even persistent pain, blood in the urine, and sometimes ulceration through tissues to form a new outlet (so called 'fistula'). The treatment depends on the site of the cancer but involves surgery or radiotherapy or both.

Cancer of the penis

This is rare in western Europe and North America but more common in the far east. The incidence is low in circumcised males. General hygiene may be a factor and a virus (HPV) has also been implicated. These tumours may present as an ulcer, usually on the glans beneath the foreskin. If it is suspected then a biopsy is essential. This is particularly important since treatment may involve surgery and even amputation of the penis. If the cancer is small a lesser operation combined with radiotherapy may be advised and in these circumstances the outlook may be excellent. Where more widespread disease is present then long-term survival is unusual.

Cancers of the testis

Cancers which start in the testes are rare, but even so they are the commonest cancers to occur in men between the ages of 20 and 35. Most of these arise in very primitive cells called 'germ cells'. Two main types of cancer can develop from these cells: a 'seminoma'—this is the commonest testis cancer and occurs predominantly between the ages

of 30 and 50 years; a 'teratoma'—these have a peak incidence between
the ages of 20 and 30.

The causes of these cancers are largely unknown although it is
recognized that the normal development of the testis involves its
descent from within the abdomen down to the scrotum and that
when this fails to happen there is a greater risk of a testis cancer
developing. Recent information suggests that teratomas are occurring
more frequently but the reasons for this are unexplained.

Presentation

The most common reason for seeking advice is painless swelling of
one testis. Inflammation of the testis (orchitis) or the tubes draining
the testis (epididymitis), both usually caused by infection, may cause
swelling but are usually painful. Occasionally the swelling may come to
notice following injury but there is no evidence whatsoever that injury
can cause a cancer. Sometimes the cancer spreads to glands within
the lower abdomen and this results in a sensation of low backache.
Enlargement of glands within the abdomen may cause swelling which
may be felt as lumps through the wall of the abdomen. Sometimes
enlarged glands may be noticed at the root of the neck. Clumps of
cancer cells reaching the lungs may cause shortness of breath.

Investigation

As for other cancers the most important investigation is a biopsy.
There is good evidence that it is better to remove the whole testis if
a diagnosis of cancer is suspected but before this is done an ultrasound
examination of both testes is now performed. Fortunately there are a
number of features which help to avoid the unnecessary removal of a
testis. The suspicion of cancer may be high from the examination but
in addition most of the cancers produce substances in the blood not
found when testis cancer is not present. These so called 'markers' (beta
HCG and alpha-fetoprotein) can be used to help both in diagnosis and
later in monitoring treatment. A simple blood test before the operation
may not only suggest that a cancer is present but also whether teratoma
or seminoma is more likely.

Once the presence of a cancer is confirmed a number of tests are
necessary to find out whether any spread has occurred and if so to

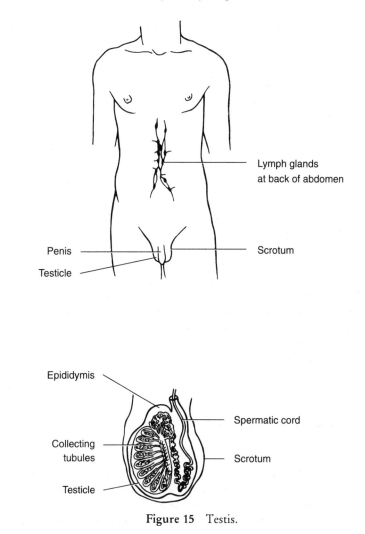

Lymph glands
at back of abdomen

Penis

Scrotum

Testicle

Epididymis

Spermatic cord

Collecting
tubules

Scrotum

Testicle

Figure 15 Testis.

where. The most valuable examination is the CT scan of the chest
and abdomen. The markers will be repeated to check that the level
has fallen with the removal of the tumour. Where a seminoma
has been diagnosed the CT scan may also help with radiotherapy
planning.

Treatment

It is now accepted that looking after someone with cancer of the testis requires special skills. Within any geographical region there is probably only one centre which can offer the comprehensive care which is likely to achieve the best results. Travel imposes strains but the period of treatment is relatively short and fortunately each treatment usually requires only three to five days in hospital.

Seminoma

The primary treatment is radiotherapy even when no disease can be shown to remain after surgery. It is given to all with the exception of those whose disease is shown to have spread more widely. Radiotherapy is highly effective and since these tumours are very sensitive the side-effects of treatment can be kept to a minimum. Fertility can often be preserved although this cannot be guaranteed.

If disease is too widespread or too bulky for radiotherapy to be given with curative intent then chemotherapy is advised. The chemotherapy used is that given for teratoma and is highly successful.

Teratoma

If the tumour has been removed and the markers and all other investigations are normal the doctor may recommend no further treatment apart from ensuring regular follow-up with measurement of markers and repeat of some scans.

The treatment of teratomas and mixed tumours (seminoma and teratoma in the same tumour) that have spread now relies almost exclusively on chemotherapy. This has transformed the outlook for most people as treatments have become more effective and side-effects have become better controlled. The choice of management and of the chemotherapy to be used depends upon the site and extent of the disease, the appearance of the tumour under the microscope and the levels of markers.

Several very active drugs are used in combination but the most important drug is called cisplatin. This has to be given by a slow drip into a vein over a period of hours. The main side-effect is nausea which is almost unavoidable but newer anti-sickness drugs mean that vomiting is much less of a problem. Hair loss affects everyone and usually becomes noticeable after three weeks or so and although it may completely affect the head hair elsewhere is often much less affected. Hair loss is only temporary and regrowth starts about two months after the chemotherapy is finished. The doctor will monitor the blood counts as these are usually lowered by treatment but recover spontaneously before the next treatment is due. He will also, at intervals, do tests to check kidney function and check the 'marker' levels in the blood. Treatment is usually planned to last a minimum of twelve weeks. If evidence of the tumour could be seen on the original CT scan this will be repeated to check that no detectable tumour remains. It is not uncommon to find that some previously abnormal areas have not quite returned to normal. If a mass can still be seen this is probably a mixture of scar tissue and normal looking cells from different tissues—a so called 'benign teratoma'. Since these can occasionally continue to grow it is normal to ask the surgeon to remove them and this also allows the pathologist to check under the microscope that no tumour remains. Once the doctor is happy that no evidence of disease remains he will want to arrange for a regular check up to be carried out and to check that sexual function is restored.

One of the greatest concerns in those who have completed treatment and who are gradually returning to normal life is whether they may be able to father children. In any debilitating illness temporary loss of sexual interest may occur but recovery is complete when the illness is over—the same is true for the period of chemotherapy. This is not usually a prolonged problem, it is however very important to seek advice if it is worrying either partner. Very occasionally hormone replacement is needed but whatever the circumstances there is nothing lost in talking over the problem with the doctor who will certainly have dealt with the problems of others. Fertility tends to be rather more of a problem as it is often reduced in men with teratoma. Fortunately the chemotherapy which is used is less likely to cause infertility than that used for some other diseases. Sperm banking prior to treatment is one way of bypassing the potential risks of chemotherapy induced infertility. It is certainly worthwhile for those who are concerned about their fertility to have a sperm examination once they have fully recovered from the treatment.

A small number of people present each year with cancers like those which occur in the testis but starting in other places. The most common site is within the chest in an area called the 'mediastinum'. This is where the heart and the main blood vessels lie between the lungs. In a minority of these people an ultrasound examination of the testes will show a small tumour there from which it is assumed the tumour spread to the chest. When this is found the affected testis is generally removed.

Prognosis

The prospect for cure for people with limited spread of their seminoma who are treated by radiotherapy is high with well over 90 per cent cured. Even the majority of those with more extensive and bulky disease can, with modern chemotherapy, anticipate cure. Most people who have a teratoma are cured by chemotherapy even when there has been spread to other parts of the body. Only a few prove to have genuinely resistant disease.

Those tumours which are found primarily in the chest tend to have a worse outlook than those which are found in the testes.

Bone cancer

The bones are a common site for primary cancer (for example breast or lung cancer) to metastasize, so most cancers in the bones are secondaries stemming from a primary elsewhere in the body. Cancers that arise as primaries in the bones are comparatively rare. It is important to distinguish between these two different forms of bone cancer as treatment options are very different; secondaries are likely to respond to the treatment that is effective for their primary 'parent' cancer.

The most common kind of primary bone cancer, making up about 40 per cent of all cases, is multiple myeloma. This is a cancer of the cells in the bone marrow, and affects the bones secondarily. As it has more in common with other haematological cancers it is discussed in a separate section on p.184.

Osteogenic sarcomas are the next most common kind of primary bone cancer (about 33 per cent of all cases). These tumours usually affect the arms or the legs near the knees. Ewing's sarcoma affects the pelvis and thigh bones. Both these cancers are more likely to affect teenagers and young adults, more often boys than girls.

Chondrosarcoma is a cancer of the cartilage, and usually affects the trunk and upper parts of the arms and legs. It is more common in middle-aged and older people, and again more often affects men than women. Approximately 13 per cent of all primary bone cancer cases are chondrosarcomas.

Malignant fibrous histiocytomas are a very rare form of bone cancer. They occur in the arms and legs, especially round the knee joint, and affect adult men and women.

Causes

The causes of primary bone cancer are generally unknown. People who have a chronic inflammatory disease of the bone (Paget's disease) have a higher risk of getting osteogenic sarcoma in their later years, but this disease affects very small numbers of people.

Secondary bone cancers are always caused by a primary cancer elsewhere in the body. Sometimes the secondary may be the first manifestation of a primary cancer that has been completely symptom-free.

Presentation

Both primary and secondary bone cancers cause pain and this is likely to be the first symptom people notice. The pain is usually deep, gnawing, and persistent, and not associated with any activity or exercise people have taken. It may keep them awake at night. Pain may, of course, be a symptom of many other conditions, but if persistent should always be checked by a doctor.

Other symptoms may include swelling or tenderness in a limb or joint (particularly in children). If the cancer has already weakened a bone, the first symptom may be a broken bone, often after a very minor fall or accident. Occasionally people experience nausea, vomiting, abdominal pain, and confusion. This occurs when a tumour causes calcium salts from the bone to dissolve into the bloodstream, raising the level of calcium in the blood (a condition called hypercalcaemia). This is particularly likely if the tumour is a secondary.

Investigations

The first diagnostic test is likely to be an X-ray. Primary bone cancers give very characteristic pictures on X-ray, showing either dark patches where the cancer has destroyed parts of the bone, or white patches where the cancer has caused deposits of extra calcium to form new bone (sclerosis). Bone scans (see p.41) are more sensitive than X-rays and can pick up very small 'hot spots' of cancer which an X-ray would not detect.

A biopsy is not usually necessary for secondary cancers, when the site of the primary is known. If there is no known primary elsewhere

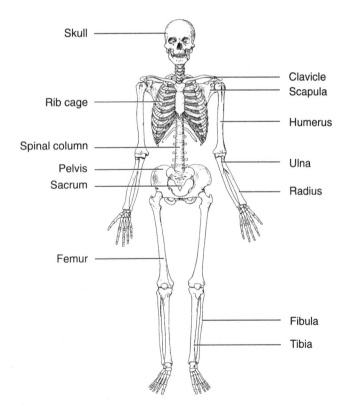

Figure 16 Bone.

in the body a biopsy is needed so that a definite diagnosis can be made by examining the cells under the microscope. Generally a needle biopsy can be taken, under a local anaesthetic. Sometimes an open biopsy is necessary, which entails an operation under general anaesthetic.

Further tests may be needed to detect whether the cancer has spread (if it is a primary) or to look for a primary (if it is a secondary and there is no known primary). Such tests would usually include a CT scan of the chest (the commonest place for primary bone cancer to metastasize), ultrasound of the liver, and sometimes MRI scans.

Treatment for primary bone cancer

Surgery is usually the first treatment for primary cancers in the bone. In the past, this almost always involved major surgery, including amputation of the affected limb. Now it is often possible to remove only the affected part of the bone and replace it with plastic, metal, or cadaver bone grafts (these newer techniques are known as limb-sparing surgery). Even if the bone cancer spreads to one or two spots on the lung, it may be possible to remove that part of the lung surgically, if the person is young and otherwise fit.

Radiotherapy is used in addition to surgery for several kinds of bone primaries. It is not usually part of the treatment for osteogenic sarcomas though may be used if for some reason an operation is not possible. Ewing's sarcoma, however, is very sensitive to radiotherapy and this treatment is often used, usually following an initial course of chemotherapy and before surgery. For chondrosarcoma, too, radiotherapy after surgery can be helpful in controlling the disease, if the tumour cannot be completely removed.

Chemotherapy too plays a useful role in treating primary tumours. It is used as adjuvant therapy after surgery for osteogenic sarcomas, to mop up any tiny metastases which may not have been removed at the operation. This has resulted in a greater number of people being cured. Recently, some doctors have been experimenting with using chemotherapy before surgery (neo-adjuvant therapy) to see if this combination improves results further. The aim is to try to shrink large tumours sufficiently to make limb-sparing surgery possible. For Ewing's sarcoma, the usual approach is to give people several cycles of chemotherapy before surgery to shrink the tumour, followed by surgery or radiotherapy or both. Chemotherapy does not play a big role in the treatment of chondrosarcoma.

Treatment for secondary bone cancer

Treatment of secondary bone tumours depends on the primary from which it comes. For example, if the primary tumour is in the breast, the secondary tumours in the bone are likely to respond to breast cancer treatments, for example hormonal therapy and chemotherapy (see p.96–98 for more details of these treatments for advanced breast cancer).

Many tumours in the bone, especially secondary tumours, activate cells in the bone called osteoclasts, which destroy the bone. Drugs called biphosphonates can be very effective in inhibiting the activity of osteoclasts, thereby slowing down and reducing the destruction of the bone.

Prognosis

Great improvements in survival rates for people with primary bone cancers have been achieved in recent years with new multidisciplinary approaches involving adjuvant and neo-adjuvant chemotherapy and radiotherapy in addition to surgery. In addition, the development of limb-sparing techniques have made surgery a less drastic treatment than in the past. It is very important that people with bone cancers should be treated in specialist cancer centres, to ensure that they receive the optimal combination of treatment for their particular disease.

Soft tissue sarcomas

Soft tissue sarcomas are cancers which affect the supporting tissues of the body—the muscle, fat, blood vessels, nerve sheaths. They are very rare, accounting for only about 1 per cent of all cancers in men and 0.6 per cent of cancers in women. A significant number, however, occur in children (for example, rhabdomyosarcomas account for between 4 and 8 per cent of all childhood tumours). There are a number of different kinds of sarcoma, depending on which kind of tissue is affected.

- **Malignant fibrous histiocytomas** are the commonest kind, and occur most often in the arms or legs, although they can affect any part of the body.

- **Fibrosarcomas** arise in the cells which make up the connective tissues of the body—the fibrocytes. These sarcomas are most commonly found in the arms, legs, or trunk.

- **Liposarcomas** are cancers that start in the fat cells, usually in the layer of fat just below the skin. These are most common in middle aged people.

- **Synovial sarcomas** occur in the synovial membrane which covers the joints in the limbs. They are more common in young adults.

- **Rhabdomyosarcomas** start in the active muscles that move joints (the biceps, for example). They occur mostly in the head, neck, and pelvis.

- **Leiomyosarcomas** occur in involuntary muscle, for example the muscles of the womb, stomach, intestine, or the blood vessels.

- **Neurofibrosarcomas** occur in the sheath that covers the nerves and can occur anywhere in the body.

Causes

The reasons why soft tissue sarcomas occur are not known. Occasionally, people who have had previous treatment with radiotherapy may develop a soft tissue sarcoma within the treated area. The use of certain wood preservatives and herbicides has come under suspicion, but no connection has been proved. Some very rare genetic diseases seem to increase the risk of getting certain sarcomas.

Presentation

The symptoms of a soft tissue sarcoma depend on where in the body the tumour has developed. If the sarcoma is in a leg or arm, the first sign will often be a swelling or lump, which may be quite hard. This is often completely painless, though occasionally such lumps will be tender.

If the sarcoma is deep in the body, it may become quite large and remain symptom-free until it begins to press on an organ or nerve. The symptoms it then produces will depend on where it is; for example a sarcoma that presses on the bowel might cause pain, vomiting, and constipation.

Investigations

The first test will be to biopsy the lump—either with a needle under local anaesthetic, or, if it is not possible to obtain sufficient tissue that way, with an open biopsy under general anaesthetic. Examination of the cells taken in this way will confirm the diagnosis.

A CT or MRI scan (see p.38) of the affected limb will enable the doctor to see accurately how large the tumour is and to plan treatment accordingly. Further tests will be done to detect any spread of the disease. For example, chest X-rays and a CT scan of the chest will detect any secondaries in the lung—a common site for soft tissue sarcomas to spread. Ultrasound of the liver will check for metastases there, and an isotope bone scan can tell whether the cancer has spread to the bone. The bone marrow may also be tested, by removing a small amount with a syringe from a hip bone.

Treatment

Combinations of surgery, radiotherapy, and sometimes chemotherapy have been used in recent years to treat soft tissue sarcomas, with greatly improved results. While surgery to remove the tumour remains the most important treatment, radiotherapy and sometimes chemotherapy are often used either before or after surgery, depending on the sensitivity of the tumour to these treatments. Soft tissue sarcomas are not easy to remove completely by surgery alone, and the combination of treatments enables doctors to treat any remaining cancer cells, thus reducing the risk of relapse.

In the past, a tumour in a limb was treated by amputation of the limb. It may still be necessary, sometimes, to remove the affected limb, but it is now often possible to remove the affected part only, by giving high doses of radiotherapy either before the operation, to shrink the tumour to make it easier to remove, or afterwards to mop up any cancer cells that have not been removed. Chemotherapy may sometimes be given before surgery to shrink the tumour and it may sometimes be possible to deliver the drugs into the artery that supplies blood to the tumour itself, thus giving higher doses directly to the tumour. Chemotherapy is being tried as adjuvant therapy after an operation, to deal with any cells that have not been removed surgically, but its use remains experimental except for tumours which are very sensitive to drug treatment.

In the case of those sarcomas which are very sensitive to chemotherapy, for example, rhabdomyosarcomas, it is sometimes possible to give very high doses of chemotherapy followed by a bone marrow or stem cell transplant.

Prognosis

With the optimal combination of treatments, results are now much improved and overall more than a third of people with a soft tissue sarcoma are cured and others have their life significantly prolonged. Improvements in surgical technique, too, have meant that treatment is less drastic, thus giving people a vastly improved quality of life.

Skin cancers

There are three major kinds of skin cancer, basal and squamous cell carcinomas and malignant melanoma. Skin cancers are one of the commonest cancers in both men and women; the first two kinds, basal and squamous cell carcinomas, make up, respectively, 75 per cent and 20 per cent of all cases of skin cancer. They are very easily detected at an early stage, and easily cured. Cases of malignant melanoma make up only 5 per cent of the total number of cases, but the incidence is rising dramatically. This kind of skin cancer is curable if it is detected at an early stage, but it is a great deal more serious than the other skin cancers. While basal cell carcinomas (also called rodent ulcers) never spread to other parts of the body, and squamous cell carcinomas do so only rarely, malignant melanoma can spread, if it is not diagnosed at an early stage.

Skin cancers are largely preventable, as they are strongly related to exposure to ultraviolet light, and damage to the skin from the sun.

The risk is greatly increased for people with fair skins; people with blond or red hair, blue eyes, and skin that freckles rather than tans are particularly at risk. Skin cancers are generally uncommon in black and Asian people. The intensity of the sunlight to which the skin is exposed also increases the risk, so fair-skinned people are at greater risk in countries near the equator than in northern Europe. Australia, which has a large population of people of northern European descent, has a very high incidence of skin cancers. As the number of hours of exposure is a significant factor, people who work outdoors or who play a lot of outdoor sports are at greater risk. There is also some suggestion that people who work indoors but take one or two holidays each year, and sunbathe in short intensive bursts may be at increased risk, particularly of melanoma.

The use of sunbeds for tanning the skin has been advertised as safe, but there is now evidence that prolonged or excessive use can increase the risk of skin cancers and melanoma. It is now suggested that sunbeds should be used in moderation, and with caution.

Protection of the skin from the sun is very important. Wearing hats, covering up with suitable clothing, avoiding the sun in the middle of the day, and using a sun protection cream with an adequate protection factor for the skin type, are all sensible preventive steps to reduce the risk, while still enjoying the sun. It is particularly important to protect children's skin from sunburn, as there is evidence to show that episodes of blistering sunburn in childhood increase susceptibility to skin cancers later in life. It is estimated that a very high proportion of most people's lifetime exposure to the sun occurs during their childhood, so ensuring children cover up, or put on a sunblock product when they go out to play, is a vital preventive step.

Most cases of skin cancer develop in older people, although melanoma can occasionally affect young people in their teens and twenties. Melanoma affects about twice as many women as men.

Presentation

Everyone has moles and small lumps on their skin. When these have remained unchanged for many years it is extremely unlikely that they are of significance. However, if an existing lump or mark changes shape, colour or size, or starts to weep or bleed it should be seen by a doctor. So too should any new lump which does not go away spontaneously in a few weeks. Most skin cancers occur in areas which are most exposed to the sun, such as the face and neck, feet and legs, and sometimes the trunk. Melanomas may, however, also occur in parts of the body which are not exposed, sometimes even on the soles of the feet. It is thought that a factor is produced by sun exposure which travels to other parts of the body in the bloodstream.

It is most important that people become aware of the changes that might indicate skin cancer, and go to their doctor as soon as they are concerned. At least 90 per cent of melanomas can be recognized at a curable stage; the mortality figures for this cancer could be greatly reduced if there were fewer delays in diagnosis.

Investigations

A suspicious skin lesion will result in referral to a skin specialist (dermatologist). Often the specialist will be able to tell when a mole or lump is not of concern by looking at it. However, if the doctor is in any doubt, a biopsy will be performed, to remove the suspect tissue surgically under a local anaesthetic and examine it under the microscope. It is usual to remove the lump entirely, so the biopsy is also the major part of the treatment. If melanoma is suspected, usually a margin of normal skin surrounding the area will be removed as well.

No further tests will be done if the cancer is a basal cell carcinoma, as these never spread to other parts of the body. Removing the lump is all that needs to be done to cure it. As it is usual for small squamous cell carcinomas to spread, there will probably be no need for further tests in this instance either.

If the cancer is malignant melanoma, the doctor will calculate the risk of its returning or spreading by assessing how deeply the cancer has penetrated into the skin, using a system called the Breslow thickness scale. If the melanoma is very thin (less than 1 mm), the risk that it has spread is very slight, and probably no further tests will be done. If, however, it has penetrated further into the skin, the risk of spread is greater, and further tests will be done, such as a chest X-ray, ultrasound of the liver, and occasionally, if symptoms indicate spread has occurred to the brain or bones, a CT scan of the head or an isotope bone scan.

Treatment

Surgery

Surgery is the major part of treatment for all skin cancers and in most cases the surgery to remove the suspect lump for diagnosis is all the treatment that is required. For basal and squamous cell carcinomas a technique called micrographic surgery is sometimes used. The surgeon removes small sections of the tumour at a time, and each section is examined under the microscope. The surgeon continues to remove tiny sections until he or she is satisfied that all the cancerous tissue has been removed. When small basal or squamous cell carcinomas appear as new small tumours after an initial diagnosis has been made, they may not be removed for diagnostic purposes and instead may be removed by electrocautery (which uses electric current to cut out and cauterize the area) or by cryosurgery (in which liquid nitrogen is used to freeze the cells which causes them to drop off).

When melanomas are operated on, an area of normal skin around the affected part is usually removed as well, to ensure that all malignant cells have been eliminated. The amount of skin that needs to be removed depends on how deeply the melanoma has penetrated into the layers of the skin. If this area is very large, plastic surgery may be needed, taking a skin graft from another part of the body to replace the tissue that has been removed. It may sometimes also be necessary to remove any lymph glands near the tumour, either to check whether or not the disease has spread, or to try to prevent further spread, if the glands seem already to be involved. Removal of the lymph glands will be done under a general anaesthetic and should not cause any disruption to normal activities afterwards. However, if the lymph glands in the armpit or groin are removed, there may be an increased risk of lymphoedema (swelling) in the limb from which the glands were taken.

Radiotherapy

Radiotherapy can be a highly effective treatment for basal and squamous cell carcinomas, as an alternative to surgery, especially in areas such as the face where surgery might cause scarring. Radiotherapy for skin cancers if very simple and has very few side-effects. The skin will be red for a few weeks and there may be a small mark left. Hair loss will only occur if the radiotherapy is directed at parts of the body which normally have hair. The hair will usually grow back once the course of radiotherapy has finished.

This treatment is not used for melanoma, which must always be surgically removed.

Chemotherapy

Chemotherapy may be used for treating skin cancers. The drugs are sometimes helpful but are still of limited value generally. Chemotherapy can cause the skin cancer to shrink in a minority of people, but cannot make it go completely, and it is not clear what effect this treatment has on prolonging life.

If the skin cancer has spread (metastasized) and the secondary cancers are causing uncomfortable or distressing symptoms, chemotherapy can sometimes shrink the metastases and thereby relieve symptoms. Occasionally, when multiple recurrences from melanoma occur in the skin of one limb, it is possible to give chemotherapy by a technique called isolated limb perfusion, which can be helpful in controlling the metastases. To do this, the blood supply to the affected limb is isolated and the drugs are put in via an artery and circulated through the limb without going through the rest of the body. In this way higher doses of chemotherapy can be given.

Other treatments

Interleukin is a natural substance which is manufactured by the body to stimulate the body's defence mechanisms against infection. It can now be manufactured by genetic engineering techniques, and is being used experimentally to treat malignant melanoma. In a minority of patients it can cause shrinkage of the tumour, but the side-effects can be severe, including fever, headaches, nausea and vomiting, weight gain, low blood pressure, skin rashes, and loss of appetite. These side-effects can be effectively controlled, and will pass after the treatment has finished, but the role of interleukin is still being evaluated.

Interferon is another treatment being used experimentally for malignant melanoma. It too is a substance normally manufactured by the body to fight viral infections, and now available for therapeutic use thanks to genetic engineering techniques. Side-effects of interferon treatment are relatively mild and similar to flu symptoms—chills, fever, joint pains, and headaches—and can be easily controlled. Interferon can help to shrink the tumours of a minority of patients.

The combination of interferon and retinoic acid (a vitamin A derivative) is being evaluated in the treatment of advanced squamous cell cancers with shrinkage of the cancer in a significant number of patients.

Hormonal treatments such as tamoxifen (an anti-oestrogen) may have a role in helping to control melanoma, possibly in combination with chemotherapy. This approach is still under evaluation.

Prognosis

Skin cancers are among the most curable of all cancers, and the overwhelming majority of people who get skin cancer are cured. Even the most serious form, malignant melanoma, is curable in the majority of cases if it is detected at an early stage. When melanomas are not detected until they have spread, cure is unlikely, and the aim of treatment is to relieve symptoms. For this reason public education programmes are vitally important—to encourage people to take sensible precautions in the sun, to make people aware of the kind of changes in a skin blemish or mole to look out for and to advise them to seek medical advice as soon as they notice any abnormalities.

Rare tumours of the skin

T cell lymphomas

Certain rare types of lymphomas have a predisposition to occur in the skin, causing skin nodules and an eczema-like rash. These conditions are known as mycosis fungoides and Sezary syndrome. As with more common low grade lymphomas (see p. 173) they respond to chemotherapy. Another technique called phototherapy has a very useful role. The patient is given a chemical which is activated by ultraviolet light and is then exposed to a source of UV light. Radiotherapy can also be useful in controlling the skin lesions.

The lymphomas

If you are reading this chapter because you or a relative or friend have a lymphoma you may be justifiably confused by anything you have so far heard. How peculiar that a group of conditions which are cancers which start in lymphoid tissues (usually in 'lymph glands' somewhere in the body) include some with a specific name (Hodgkin's disease—HD) and all the rest are called 'non'-somethings (non-Hodgkin lymphomas—NHL). The logic for this (which is pretty thin) is that the clinical behaviour of Hodgkin's disease, for the most part, follows a fairly predictable pattern whereas the remainder of the lymphomas are very different in character and behaviour and are therefore labelled as non-Hodgkin lymphomas. In fact modern pathological techniques allow us to recognize many varieties of lymphoma and occasionally distinctions between some types of Hodgkin's disease and non-Hodgkin lymphomas may not be possible with absolute certainty. For the most part it is possible to label a lymphoma either as Hodgkin's disease or a non-Hodgkin lymphoma and as there are subtypes of each it is this along with other investigations which will influence treatment and give some idea of future outlook. The good management of these conditions requires a highly professional approach which needs the resources normally found only in cancer centres.

Hodgkin's disease

This was first described in 1835 but some of the cases used to illustrate this condition would not now be called HD. It is uncommon, having an incidence of about 3/100 000, is slightly more common in males than females, and is found most commonly between 10 and 25 years of age. There is a lower incidence until about 50 when there is a slow rise which peaks around 70 years of age.

Causes

No cause has yet been identified although there is a suspicion that the virus which causes glandular fever (Epstein–Barr virus) may somehow be involved. Since glandular fever is common in young adults and Hodgkin's disease is very rare the connection must depend on other very unusual characteristics or events which have yet to be identified.

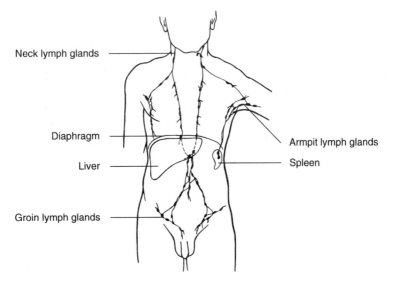

Figure 17 The lymph glands.

Genetic and environmental factors cannot be ruled out for more than one family member in the same or different generations may be affected, and in identical twins the risk of the second twin developing Hodgkin's disease after the first is diagnosed is very high. There have been reports of clusters of cases being found in a community but these are not common and may be due entirely to chance.

Presentation

Commonly Hodgkin's disease first declares as painless enlargement of lymph glands. Glands which enlarge in the neck as a result of a severe sore throat are often modest in size, affect both sides of the neck, and are tender. In Hodgkin's disease the glands may appear in one or more sites where glands are found such as different regions of the neck, the armpits, or the groin. They persist longer than would be the case if there was a straightforward infection and slowly enlarge. In some people the glands may have been present for months before they decide to see a doctor. Many people do not have any particular symptoms but in about a third of cases so called 'B symptoms' occur. These may be night sweats, which may be severe enough to need a change of sheets, weight loss (which to be significant must be greater than 10 per cent of the body weight within a six month period), or both. Other symptoms which are well recognized but which do not count as B symptoms are generalized itching which may be severe and does not resolve until the Hodgkin's disease is treated and 'alcohol pain'. This is discomfort felt in the glands or other areas involved by Hodgkin's disease which comes on almost immediately after drinking alcohol. Although uncommon, this can occasionally be useful in suggesting that the Hodgkin's disease has recurred in someone who experienced these symptoms initially.

Investigations

No diagnosis of lymphoma can be made without the examination of suspect tissue under the microscope. The usual way to obtain this is by 'biopsy' removal of a whole enlarged gland. Several types of Hodgkin's disease are recognized but the commonest by far (80–90 per cent) is called 'nodular sclerosing' followed by 'mixed cellularity'. Rare subtypes are 'lymphocyte predominant' (generally carries a better than usual prognosis) and 'lymphocyte depleted' (tends to occur in older people and to be harder to control).

A feature of Hodgkin's disease which distinguishes it from the non-Hodgkin lymphomas is that it appears to start in one lymph node group (such as, low in the neck) and spread to the group next door (such as, higher in the neck). The doctor will therefore feel very carefully to see whether he can find any enlarged glands in the sites where glands do occur. These include both sides of the neck, both back and front; above and below the clavicles; the armpits; just above the elbows and the groin. He will also feel the abdomen on the right hand side to see whether the liver is enlarged, on the left to feel for the spleen (which is full of lymphoid tissue and therefore like a big lymph gland) and elsewhere in case any of the deep glands in the abdomen are large enough to be felt.

The preliminary examination gives a clue as to how extensive the disease might be but not nearly enough information on which to base treatment which is why a number of additional tests are needed. These are often called 'staging investigations' because they help to define the extent or 'stage' of the disease. Inevitably there are blood tests to check for blood cell production, for evidence of inflammation and that the kidneys and liver are working normally. Blood tests will also be done to check the levels of the proteins and the cells involved in immunity. A chest X-ray is vital since the glands in the middle of the chest are sometimes enlarged, indeed very occasionally this is the only site of Hodgkin's disease. The abdomen can now be assessed using a CT scanner and this shows up enlarged glands, even those deep within the abdomen alongside the aorta. Some years ago the only way to examine this area well was by operation—a major procedure during which the spleen was also removed, but this approach has now been abandoned. A CT scan of the chest is carried out at the same time as the abdominal examination as this allows a very close look at the 'mediastinum', the middle of the chest where Hodgkin's disease is sometimes found even when the chest X-ray is normal. A bone marrow examination is carried out if it is felt that there is a possibility that this might be involved by Hodgkin's disease since the treatment would need to be tailored to treat this effectively.

Once all these results are available the extent of the disease will be categorized using the so called Ann Arbor classification, named after the town in the USA where the medical meeting at which the scheme was devised took place. It is quite useful to know the outline of this scheme since it is widely used.

- Stage I—involvement of a single lymph node site.

- Stage II—involvement of two or more lymph node sites on the same side of the diaphragm.

- Stage III—involvement of lymph node sites on both sides of the diaphragm (the spleen is regarded here as a lymph node).

- Stage IV—diffuse involvement of one or more organs (such as bone marrow or liver) with or without gland involvement.

Those who do not have the 'B symptoms' described earlier are sub-categorized 'A'. For example someone who has glands in the left neck only and no symptoms has IA disease, and someone with disease involving the bone marrow and B symptoms has IVB disease.

Treatment

Nowadays doctors at most centres have organized themselves into teams and a great deal of consultation and discussion will take place as the investigations proceed in order to decide on the best approach to treatment.

Radiotherapy

The staging system described above is widely used as a way of selecting treatments on a logical basis. Local treatment with radiotherapy makes very good sense if the disease is low volume and likely to be localized (IA and IIA). The presence of 'B' symptoms makes localized disease unlikely and radiotherapy is now never used as primary treatment in someone who has these symptoms. However, Hodgkin's disease is very sensitive to radiotherapy and where it is confined to lymph glands in discrete groups on the same side of the diaphragm then this is the treatment of choice. Since no tests are wholly reliable in defining the spread of Hodgkin's disease a decision which the radiotherapist has to take is how big an area to treat in order not to miss disease which might be at the margins. The sub-type may be helpful here—for example, some types of 'lymphocyte predominant' Hodgkin's disease are almost always localized so that only a small area need be treated. In most cases treatment is given for localized disease above the diaphragm to a so called 'mantle' area which extends from the base of the skull down to just below the diaphragm. This takes in all the gland areas of the neck, both armpits, and the glands in the centre of the chest. As the lungs come into this area they are protected during treatments by lead shielding. Each treatment lasts only a few minutes in each day but is repeated 4 to 5 days in each week over several weeks. This division of the total radiation dose is called 'fractionation' and is a way of reducing radiation damage to the normal tissues.

A similar approach is taken to disease below the diaphragm (IA and IIA) but here treatment has to include the spleen. Any radiotherapy to a relatively large area has some general side-effects, in particular tiredness and lethargy. Some people may become temporarily depressed. Where the bowel is included in the field some bowel upset is almost inevitable. Medical and nursing teams are better than ever at helping with such problems although at times these may be temporarily difficult to keep in check. Once the treatment is completed recovery begins and side-effects should gradually resolve.

A special problem concerns bulky glands especially when these are in the chest. Radiotherapy would have to include a large volume of lung and risk permanent damage. For this reason chemotherapy is given first in order to shrink down the glands; radiotherapy can then be given to a normal sized field and further chemotherapy follows with the intent of eradicating any disease which might remain.

Chemotherapy

Combinations of certain anti-cancer drugs have been shown to be highly effective at treating Hodgkin's disease even when it is quite widespread. It is therefore important to realize that the choice of chemo-therapy as the main treatment is not a second best. The various regimens have different acronyms based on the drug names. The oldest and best known of these is MOPP (mustine, Oncovin/vincristine, procarbazine, and prednisolone) but as mustine has a number of unpleasant side-effects this has been replaced by chlorambucil and the vincristine by v(inblastine) to make ChVPP. Another well tried combination is a(driamycin), b(leomycin), v(inblastine), d(TIC). New ways of giving these treatments have led to shorter duration of treatments and a reduc-tion of side-effects. An example of this is p(rednisolone), a(driamycin), c(yclophosphamide), e(toposide) which is given on alternate weeks with b(leomycin), O(ncovin/vincristine), m(ethotrexate) in the inter-vening weeks. These treatments require attendance at the oncology unit for most of the drugs are given into a vein. Side-effects are less of a problem than they used to be but require close supervision to keep these at a minimum. Nausea and sickness can be minimized, but effects on the blood count require careful supervision. Hair loss occurs with some regimens and not others and once treatment is complete the hair grows back.

While it is likely that most of these regimens are equally effective, clinical trials continue to play an important role in refining these treatments and therefore will often be discussed prior to treatment.

The Hodgkin's disease is not going away or has come back

It is unusual for Hodgkin's disease not to respond to treatment and if it does not go away other varieties of treatment have to be considered. This may include high dose therapy and stem cell or bone marrow transplantation or support (see p.62–68). However, 'complete remission' is the normal outcome of the treatments outlined earlier. This means that however hard one looks it is not possible to find any evidence of

Hodgkin's disease. In the event of the disease recurring (and a biopsy is usually essential to prove this) some of the initial investigations will be repeated. The choice of treatment will depend on a number of factors including the initial treatment, the interval since the first treatment was completed, the site(s) of the recurrence, and whether or not symptoms are present. Although the results of treatment are not as successful second time round it is still possible to achieve a complete remission and in some people this means that the disease will not come back.

Long-term side-effects of treatment

Most of the treatments given for Hodgkin's disease are remarkably free of long-term side-effects. For those treated during the reproductive age the possibility of infertility following chemotherapy has for some been a great concern. While sperm banking may get round this it is not a solution. Fertility is almost certainly reduced in many prior to treatment (sperm examination often indicates this) MOPP causes almost total sterility in men and a substantial reduction in fertility in women. An attraction of regimens such as ABVD and PACE-BOM are that they are much less sterilizing.

Second cancers, that is different kinds of cancer, appear to be an identifiable risk in those who have received a great deal of treatment with both radiotherapy and chemotherapy over a prolonged period of time. The risk is very small relative to the risk from Hodgkin's disease if it is not treated effectively. Modern chemotherapy or radiotherapy alone appear associated with a substantially lesser risk.

Follow-up

It is common to see people who have completed their treatment at fairly frequent intervals for the first few years in order to ensure that life and the consequences of Hodgkin's disease and its treatment are returning to normal. These visits should be used as an opportunity to deal with any queries which might arise, eventually minimizing the significance of Hodgkin's disease so that like any other illness it is one from which the individual has completely recovered. There are some sensible precautions which are likely to have been advised: those who have had their spleen removed or irradiated are slightly more at risk from bacterial infection by 'pneumococcus' which can cause pneumonia or even a life threatening infection. Immunization is therefore recommended. Although it is difficult to demonstrate that immunity is diminished it is thought wise to avoid immunization with live vaccines, certainly for a few years following treatment.

Prognosis

More than half of the people treated for Hodgkin's disease will be cured and for many others prolonged good quality life will be possible. Failure to eradicate the disease despite appropriate treatment or early recurrence cause understandable concern but even so some people live with chronic Hodgkin's disease for prolonged periods.

The non-Hodgkin lymphomas

Much of what has been written about Hodgkin's disease also applies to the non-Hodgkin lymphomas (NHL), but there are very important differences and these will be emphasized. For example the NHL are a group of conditions that behave very differently from one another. Overall they have a greater tendency to spread (in particular to blood forming tissues) than does Hodgkin's disease. They also are more common with increasing age and the incidence (around 7–8/100 000) in the population is greater and appears to be rising.

Causes

No definite causes have been identified. In Africa but not in Europe the very common virus associated with glandular fever appears to have some role in the development of a rare lymphoma, now known as 'Burkitt's lymphoma', after a surgeon named Denis Burkitt who first recognized the possible association.

A number of very rare medical conditions are associated with a higher than normal risk of developing NHL. Recently lymphomas have been identified as a significant consequence of AIDS and these have proved especially difficult to control even with modern treatments.

Presentation

Like Hodgkin's disease the NHL may present as persistent swelling of lymph glands but many more groups of glands may be involved. The glands may be quite small or occasionally some groups may have grown to be quite large in a relatively short time. A feature of NHL which is quite unlike Hodgkin's disease is that tissues other than lymph glands, such as bowel, the testes, skin, and occasionally the nervous system may be involved. This is more often a feature of those lymphomas which behave in a more aggressive way for the spectrum of behaviour of the NHL varies from a disease which waxes and wanes over many years to one which appears in a matter of days and may cause problems and even death within a week or so. Happily the latter is uncommon and curiously it is a group of the aggressive lymphomas which may even be cured by chemotherapy. Symptoms of night sweats, fevers, weight loss, and malaise also occur in those with NHL as in those with Hodgkin's disease.

Diagnosis and investigation

This has to be made by examining some of the suspect tissue which has been removed (a gland, or wedge of tissue, or bone marrow, etc., or examination of the tumour specimen removed at operation) under the microscope. This, as in the case of Hodgkin's disease, needs to be seen by a pathologist with special expertise in the lymphomas as interpretation may be quite difficult. Many sub-types are recognized and although some of these do not appear at the moment to have much relevance in making treatment more precise they will probably help us to understand the disease better.

The fact that there are three major classifications of the pathology in use gives a clue to the difficulties faced by pathologists. There are three main categories of NHL (although even these are slightly different in each classification):

- LOW GRADE: Long natural history (months or years) even when widespread (they commonly are—many involve the bone marrow)

- INTERMEDIATE GRADE: Shorter natural history (weeks or months) and often more localized

- HIGH GRADE: Short natural history (days or weeks) usually widespread.

The investigations are similar to those for Hodgkin's disease and are designed to determine the extent of the disease. The staging system is the same but since the NHL appear to spread both by direct growth into neighbouring structures and via the blood stream it is much less helpful. Involvement of the nervous system can occur in intermediate and high grade lymphomas and if suspected this will need special investigations.

Treatment

This will be planned by the lymphoma team on the basis of the results of the staging investigations and will be influenced by a number of factors including: the type of lymphoma; the sites of the disease; whether or not it is bulky; whether there are other medical complications.

1. LOW GRADE: A tiny number of patients have truly localized low grade lymphomas and these can be treated with local radiotherapy. In some of these the lymphoma will never recur but by and large low grade lymphomas are not curable with any currently available treatment.

Very often the process is so indolent that no treatment is required immediately—glands can wax and wane in size and if the glands become persistently larger may only require several courses of tablet treatment. This treatment (usually with 'chlorambucil') is given to those with symptoms or bulky glands at the outset and can be repeated many times. The intervals between treatments may be months in some people and even years in others. The main side-effects of chlorambucil are on the blood counts with occasional people suffering nausea. Very rarely skin rashes occur and when this happens a different drug has to be used. If tablet treatment alone is not proving effective then combination drug treatments are used as in the intermediate grade lymphomas (see below). Occasionally radiotherapy is used to control a group of glands if they are particularly troublesome. A new drug called Fludarabine is increasingly being used as second line treatment and seems likely to be useful.

2. INTERMEDIATE GRADE: Combination drug therapy is the main treatment for this group of lymphomas. The best known is called 'CHOP' which combines: cyclophosphamide, doxorubicin, vincristine, and prednisolone. The main side-effects are nausea at the time of injection, depression of the blood counts, and hair loss. The hair loss is temporary and regrowth begins about two months after treatment is completed. This can usually be given as an out-patient and only requires admission to hospital if there is a suggestion of an infection when the blood counts are low. Many other drug combinations have been tried but although some are as good as CHOP none seem better. More than half of those treated will lose all detectable evidence of disease and evidence now shows that about half of these will remain free from recurrence of lymphoma. If the disease does come back alternative drug combinations or high dose therapy with stem cell or bone marrow support (p.62–68) may be used.

3. HIGH GRADE LYMPHOMAS: these include lymphoblastic and 'Burkitt-like' lymphomas and are managed with chemotherapy similar to that for intermediate lymphomas but given more intensively. This requires admission to hospital with special attention to speedy treatment should there be a suggestion of infection when the white count is low. There is quite a high risk of involvement of the nervous system so that during the treatment programme injections of an anti-cancer drug are given into the fluid around the spinal cord and brain in order to try to prevent this. These diseases tend to be very sensitive to chemotherapy and 'melt away' but also risk coming back just as quickly so that other treatments including high dose therapy with stem cell or bone marrow support (p.62–68) are now considered.

Follow-up

After treatment is completed it is sensible to be reassured that all is either returning to normal or is at least stable. Many people with persisting NHL can anticipate living for many years and so have to learn to live with their disease just as a diabetic lives with theirs. For this reason appointments are arranged at fairly frequent intervals in the first instance so that both the doctor and the patient can learn how the disease is behaving and deal with any problems, should they occur, to minimize their importance. Research developments in the lymphomas are happening all the time with experimental approaches to developing antibody treatments with and without new drugs. Visits to outpatients are a useful way of putting these in a rather better perspective than is achieved by reading most less well informed reports. Many centres will be engaged in their own research or closely linked to that of others and will be keen for their own patients to be the first to benefit from sound developments.

Prognosis

Low grade lymphomas are rarely cured unless they are truly localized and this is fairly rare, but even so most behave chronically and are compatible with many years good quality life. Surprisingly about a third of some of the more aggressive lymphomas (the intermediate or 'diffuse large cell lymphomas') can be cured. The results of treating the high grade lymphomas are less good.

Multiple myeloma

This condition is more common in the elderly but even so, remains remarkably rare. It is best described as the cancer of the cells which produce antibodies ('plasma cells'). Normally these cells, which are related to lymphocytes, have a very important role in enforcing immunity to certain infections. The proteins produced by these cells are called immunoglobulins and they have a particular shape and structure which is directly related to substances produced by bacteria, viruses, and fungi against which the cells have been 'immunized' so protecting against infection. Myeloma is characterized by a single population of these cells producing a specific protein which can be measured in the blood or, occasionally, in the urine.

This is one of the conditions which was found to be increased in survivors of the atomic bomb explosions in Japan, although an increased incidence was not apparent until twenty or more years afterwards. The commonest site for myeloma cells to develop is in the bone marrow where plasma cells are mixed in with the normal blood-forming tissues. The myeloma cells may divide and multiply and in doing so squeeze out the normal blood forming elements. This may result in anaemia, a fall in the number of white cells in the blood, and also sometimes of the particles in the blood which prevent bruising and bleeding (called platelets). If this happens the main symptoms will be those of anaemia, such as shortness of breath, palpitations, and pallor. Bruising is less common. Occasionally, the myeloma cells multiply at one point within the bone marrow and expand locally in such a way that the bone is affected at that site. This may cause pain and if the process continues for long enough, may even weaken the bone enough to result in a fracture.

Since the abnormal proteins produced by these cells are not useful in protecting against infections antibodies may not be produced and an infection may actually be the problem which leads to the diagnosis being made. Very rarely, kidney damage may be caused by the myeloma protein. Often the symptoms resulting from the myeloma are much more subtle and it is only after a number of diagnostic tests are carried out that a diagnosis of myeloma is suspected.

Myeloma may vary in its presentation from a solitary clump of tissue with little or no production of abnormal immunoglobulin, to a widespread disease involving bone marrow and bones causing anaemia and depression of the normal bone marrow producing tissues.

Diagnosis

Although the doctor may ask a variety of questions which lead to a suspicion of anaemia and a range of conditions which might include myeloma, the diagnosis can only be made after a number of tests have been carried out. The important ones include: a blood test, to check whether anaemia is present, and whether the normal blood elements are depressed in any way; tests for kidney function because of the risks of damage by the myeloma proteins; a special blood test to determine whether the antibody proteins (immunoglobulins) are present in normal amounts. In myeloma, one sub-class of the immunoglobulins is usually raised, while the others may be depressed. A 24-hour collection of urine is usually requested in order to try to detect very tiny amounts of fragments of the immunoglobulins. This is called 'Bence Jones protein' and if present at all it is usually in such small amounts that the urine collected over 24 hours has to be concentrated to detect it. It is usual to carry out an X-ray examination of a number of bones of the body. The skull is included in this examination since myeloma in some people produces a particularly recognizable effect on skull bones.

Although a diagnosis can often be made on these tests alone, examination of the bone marrow may reveal increased numbers of the cells responsible for myeloma. Very occasionally a soft tissue collection of myeloma cells—a plasmacytoma—occurs and this may be the only evidence of disease.

Treatment

A wide range of different drugs have been tried in myeloma. One of the most successful of these is a drug called melphalan which can be given in tablet form. This is often given with prednisolone (a relative of cortisone). Melphalan tablets are often given as five to seven day courses at six weekly intervals and although there is not usually a dramatic effect on the myeloma, in those whose disease is sensitive to melphalan, abnormal protein levels in the blood gradually fall and the symptoms begin to diminish. If there are abnormal areas on X-ray these can, after a period of months, be seen to improve. For the occasional solitary lesion in bone, or one which is particularly painful, radiotherapy given either as a solitary treatment, or over a period of a few days, may produce great relief, and eventual healing. Some newer treatments including drug combinations have been used and while there is a suggestion that these may be more effective than tablets alone at getting rid of detectable disease in the short term the impact on long-term survival is not yet clear. Approaches which include high-dose chemotherapy in combination with autologous bone marrow or stem cell support are being looked at in clinical trials (see p.62–68). Although the results of some of these trials look encouraging the long-term benefits have still to be established so that high dose treatment has not yet become a routine. Interferon has some activity against myeloma cells and is being used in some centres to try to improve the long-term control of the disease.

Prognosis

In people whose disease is causing virtually no symptoms and which appears to change very little over the course of time and in those whose disease appears to be well controlled by treatment, good quality life may be achieved for a matter of years. The outlook is less good in those with symptoms or where treatment does not seem to be effective.

Waldenstron's macroglobulinaemia

Unlike myeloma this condition hardly ever affects bone. It is commonly associated with enlarged lymph glands and enlargement of the liver and spleen. One particular sub-type of antibody protein (immunoglobulin) is raised in this condition, and sometimes can rise to such high levels that the sluggishness caused to the blood flow produces symptoms which include confusion, headache, disturbances of blood clotting, and kidney function. This condition is usually treated with a drug similar in action to melphalan called chlorambucil which is often given with prednisolone. Good responses do occur and may last for months or years at a time. This condition has a rather better outlook than myeloma.

The leukaemias

These are rare cancers which develop in one of the types of white cells in the blood. The names can be very confusing but are in fact very straightforward when the system is understood. Those arising in lymphoid cells (the cells concerned with immunity) are called after the appearance of the cells under the microscope. If the cells only mature so far these may look like lymphoid cells in the early stages of development—so called 'lymphoblasts' and since the growth of these cells tends to be rather active the illness is usually rapid in onset, it is therefore called 'acute lymphoblastic leukaemia'. Where the cells develop to look almost like normal mature lymphocytes the course of the disease tends to be more sedate and is called 'chronic lymphocytic leukaemia'. The same principles apply to the leukaemias which develop in the white cells which protect against infection (the granulocytes or neutrophils). Where the cells stay in their very young state these are called 'myeloblasts' and as the process is usually aggressive and the course of the untreated disease short it is called 'acute' myeloblastic leukaemia. Where the cells mature to resemble normal adult cells (the granulocytes) the resulting illness is usually much less acute than acute myeloblastic leukaemia and is called 'chronic granulocytic leukaemia'. This form of leukaemia although described as chronic is often more aggressive in its behaviour than chronic lymphocytic leukaemia which in some people may not require treatment for a decade or more.

Acute lymphoblastic leukaemia (ALL) is the most common leukaemia of childhood with a peak incidence below the age of 10, this then declines and the incidence once again increases over the age of 50. Acute myeloblastic leukaemia (AML) is rare in childhood but has an increasing incidence with age. It is the commoner acute leukaemia in adults.

Genetic abnormalities, radiation, certain chemicals, and viruses have been implicated in the causation of some leukaemias. The survivors of the atomic bombs in Japan, particularly those near to the centres of the explosions, had an increased incidence of AML and of chronic granulocytic leukaemia. This was particularly apparent in the five year period which began two years after the bombs were dropped. AML is seen in more people treated with both radiotherapy and chemotherapy for Hodgkin's disease than in those treated with either radiotherapy or chemotherapy alone. Exposure to benzene has long been recognized to be associated with an increased risk of AML and rare variants of ALL occurring in the Caribbean and Japan have been linked to infection by a specific virus. Some very rare conditions caused by genetic abnormalities also carry an increased risk of leukaemia, among these is Down's syndrome in which ALL occurs more commonly than might be expected.

There are several sub-types of the acute leukaemias but these will be dealt with collectively under the heading of AML and ALL for the management principles are very similar.

Presentation

In both AML and ALL the large numbers of primitive cells in the blood and bone marrow may compromise the formation of the normal blood cells. Anaemia (shortage of red blood cells) can cause shortness of breath, tiredness, weakness, and pallor. A shortage of the cells which protect against infection (the neutrophils or granulocytes) may be suspected because infections are more serious or persist for longer than would normally be expected. Tiny particles in the blood called

some children with ALL the disease will not recur, unfortunately this is rarely true for adults with either AML or ALL. Continuation of some anti-leukaemic drugs after complete remission has been obtained appears useful in ALL but has not been shown to increase survival significantly in AML.

In an attempt to reduce the risk of relapse bone marrow transplantation (using donor bone marrow—preferably from a genetically similar relative) is now being considered for certain people, in particular those at high risk of relapse. Bone marrow transplantation is not without risk but supportive care has become very skilful and the results both of conventional therapy for acute leukaemia and of bone marrow transplantation continue to improve. In comparing the results it is very important to remember that although the results of bone marrow transplantation may look quite encouraging you are looking at a very carefully selected group of people who are not at all representative of all those who get acute leukaemia. The doctor explaining bone marrow transplantation will be very ready to discuss every aspect of the treatment on more than one occasion if necessary. More recently autologous bone marrow or stem cell support is being tried (see p.62–68).

Once the leukaemia recurs after a complete remission it is usually difficult to control for any length of time. The same principles of treatment apply. If the complete remission has lasted some years it is possible that the original treatment may again be successful. Great care will be taken to explain and to discuss the objectives of treatment. Although complete remission is again the aim, if this is not quickly obtained it may be better to try to deal with important symptoms rather than make matters worse by continuing to give anti-leukaemia drugs which are not proving effective but still produce unwanted side-effects. This can be a frightening realization but should be discussed fully with the doctors concerned. In major centres experimental drugs are often available—they are used as part of a carefully devised research protocol and their possible value can be explained to those who are interested.

The chronic leukaemias

Like the acute leukaemias these occur primarily in lymphoid cells (chronic lymphocytic leukaemia—CLL) or in the white cells of the bone marrow forming the granulocytes (chronic granulocytic leukaemia—CGL). Both while rare have an increasing incidence with age although CGL is found more commonly in middle age than CLL.

Chronic granulocytic leukaemia

This disease as its name implies begins more gradually than the acute leukaemias but because the bone marrow is compromised in the same way many of the symptoms are similar. Constitutional symptoms, that is general symptoms of being unwell are more common and these include loss of weight and malaise. As the spleen is frequently enlarged discomfort in the upper left part of the abdomen is common and sometimes may be severe. This may give rise to a feeling of fullness in the stomach particularly after meals and may contribute to the weight loss by causing loss of appetite. Occasionally the disease is diagnosed in the absence of symptoms following a blood count at a routine medical examination, but this is unusual.

Investigation

The blood test usually shows a very high white blood count. Occasionally there is a mild anaemia but the platelet count may be raised as the bone marrow behaves in an overactive fashion. A bone marrow examination often shows this overactive state but little else. The diagnostic features are the blood count, a special test measuring an enzyme in the white cells (the leucocyte alkaline phosphatase—this is low or absent), and the appearance in 80 per cent of people of an absolutely classical chromosome abnormality, the so-called Philadelphia chromosome. Where it is present this chromosome is a marker for the disease process and newer treatments therefore concentrate on trying to eliminate it.

Treatment

There are several useful drugs available and most can be given by mouth so that treatment can be administered as an out-patient. The most commonly used is busulphan. This drug has a powerful effect on the white count so that the doctor will ask for fairly frequent blood counts. Initially the drug allopurinol will also be given to reduce the risk of uric acid crystals (formed from the products of rapidly breaking down cells) damaging the kidney. Once the white count is down to a near normal level treatment will be discontinued and the blood counts will then be monitored at regular intervals. Re-treatment is always necessary after an interval which varies from one individual to another and eventually a change of treatment may be necessary to control the white count satisfactorily. Because the spleen is a major site of the disease and often the main source of symptoms local radiotherapy to the spleen may be considered to control pain as may surgical removal. Neither of these procedures has an influence on survival but may be useful for symptom control.

The natural history of this disease is of increasing resistance to treatment and then eventually of transformation to a disease very like acute myeloblastic leukaemia which is extremely resistant to available treatments. Newer approaches to treatment are therefore beginning to focus on ways of delaying or preventing this transformation. Bone marrow transplantation is of particular interest as in some cases it is possible to eliminate the Philadelphia chromosome although it is as yet uncertain whether this is permanent.

Chronic lymphocytic leukaemia

This is found predominantly in the elderly and may be a chance finding on a blood count in someone who is otherwise well and symptom free. In most people who have chronic lymphocytic leukaemia there is evidence of enlargement of the lymph glands, the spleen, and sometimes the liver. This may be very discrete or occasionally the glands can be quite large, even enough to cause someone to see their doctor because the swellings have become unsightly.

In most people this is a very indolent condition compatible with many years of normal life and only in the later stages of the illness does the crowding of the bone marrow by the leukaemic lymphocytes begin to compromise the production of the normal cells. When this happens anaemia may result and eventually also an increased risk of bruising and bleeding. Since the leukaemic process involves cells which are normally concerned with immunity an increased susceptibility to infections is common and occasionally bacteria, viruses, and fungus infections are difficult to eradicate.

The diagnosis is often made on a blood count alone but occasionally a lymph gland is removed if more information is required. No treatment at all may be necessary but if the glands are large or uncomfortable, if there are any symptoms or if anaemia is a problem tablet treatment may be given with cyclophosphamide or chlorambucil. Prednisolone, a more powerful form of cortisone, may also be given as this can be helpful and does not depress the blood counts. Where these have become less effective fludarabine is sometimes tried. Very occasionally radiotherapy is used to treat a group of glands if these are troublesome.

Prognosis

Chronic lymphocytic leukaemia is usually very chronic in its behaviour and since it occurs predominantly in later life some people can expect to live out their lifespan and die of so called natural causes. In younger people although it may shorten life expectancy the majority can expect to live a good quality life for a number of years.

Chronic granulocytic leukaemia tends to behave more aggressively and usually needs treatment which is why there is increasing interest in bone marrow transplantation. The outlook is less good than for chronic lymphocytic leukaemia.

Hairy cell leukaemia

This extraordinary name is given to a very rare form of leukaemia because of the microscopic appearance of the cells. They have hairy protuberances on their surface (which can only be seen under the microscope). It rarely causes enlargement of the lymph glands but because it involves the bone marrow may cause anaemia and susceptibility to infection. The spleen is often enlarged and its removal does seem to be helpful in stabilizing the condition in some people with an improvement in the blood count after the operation. Chemotherapy is of little value but interferon has been used to good effect in a proportion of those treated. It seems to have an indolent course with good quality life being possible over a matter of years for many.

Childhood tumours

The outlook for children who have cancer has changed beyond all recognition over the last twenty to thirty years, thanks to improved regimens combining surgery, radiotherapy, and chemotherapy in optimal ways. Before the 1960s, prospects for cure were poor, but cure rates have been rising steadily for all kinds of cancers that affect children, and especially dramatically for some leukaemias and lymphomas. Figures from America for all childhood cancers show a rise in five-year survival rate from 28 per cent in the period 1960–3 to 65.2 per cent in 1980–5. These figures continue to improve.

Slightly less than half of all cancers to affect children are haematological cancers—leukaemias and lymphomas—which are discussed on p.173–194. Brain tumours, which are discussed on p.78–82, are the commonest solid tumour, overall, and bone cancer and soft tissue sarcomas are also relatively common (see p.160–171). This chapter will discuss three other major tumours which are relatively common in children: neuroblastoma, Wilm's tumour, and retinoblastoma.

Neuroblastoma

This is a comparatively common cancer in children, after brain tumours and the leukaemias and lymphomas. It is a cancer of primitive tissue which evolves into part of the nervous system. It usually occurs in younger children, under the age of two years.

Presentation

The most usual symptom is a lump, often in the abdomen, chest, or neck. Frequently the child will be generally unwell, perhaps lethargic and feverish. Often the cancer will have existed for some time before producing symptoms, and at the time of diagnosis most children have quite widespread disease, which may have spread to the bone, bone marrow, liver, or brain.

Investigations

Ultrasound, CT, MRI, and isotope bone scans may all be performed (see p.38–41) to investigate the lump, check its extent, and also to detect any spread. Neuroblastomas secrete a chemical called vanillylmandelic acid (VMA) and it is often possible to detect this in the blood or urine, so blood and urine testing will be performed. A bone marrow examination is always done to check whether there is any tumour in the bone marrow, and a biopsy of the lump, under general anaesthetic, may be necessary to confirm the diagnosis if the other tests suggest a strong likelihood of a neuroblastoma.

Treatment

If the tumour is localized and has not spread to other parts of the body, surgery to remove it completely offers the best chance of cure. Neuroblastomas are very sensitive to chemotherapy and radiotherapy, and if the disease has spread beyond the original site, they may be used singly or in combination. Sometimes, too, chemotherapy or radiotherapy may be given before surgery to shrink the tumour to make it operable. Very high doses of chemotherapy may sometimes be given, followed by a bone marrow transplant (see p.62–68), when the disease has spread widely and conventional treatment doses are insufficient to deal with it. Treatment with a radioactive substance attached to a special chemical called MIBG, which is taken up by neuroblastoma cells, may also be given. This substance is given by injection into a vein. The child is mildly radioactive for a few days and will be kept in hospital during that time (see p.47 for more details about this kind of treatment). This treatment has very few side-effects.

Prognosis

One very interesting aspect of neuroblastomas is that some children, particularly under the age of one, undergo spontaneous remission of their cancer without any treatment. In addition, children under one, even if their disease is widespread, generally have a better chance of survival than older children.

The overall cure rate for children with a localized tumour that can be removed surgically is about 84 per cent. For children who have advanced disease, the cure rate is lower. However, advances in treatment, and techniques such as bone marrow transplantation mean that the outlook for these children can continue to improve too.

Wilms' tumour (nephroblastoma)

This is a less common tumour than neuroblastoma and, like neuroblastoma, it is a cancer of primitive tissues, in this case those that lie within the kidney. It develops in children between the ages of two and five, and occurs equally in boys and girls. Rarely it can occur in teenagers and adults. There is a genetic element to the development of the disease and in very small numbers of cases the children carry a genetic abnormality.

Presentation

The most usual symptom is a lump in the abdomen while the child seems otherwise entirely well. Occasionally the child may have pain in the abdomen or blood in the urine, or feel generally unwell (though this is not as common as with neuroblastoma). The tumour may spread to other parts of the body such as the lung, liver, brain, and bones, and cause symptoms in those sites.

Investigations

An ultrasound scan of the abdomen is likely to be the first test to give a clear picture of the swelling. A CT scan (see p.38) can enable the doctor to visualize the kidneys more clearly. A biopsy of the mass will be done under general anaesthetic for examination under a microscope to confirm the diagnosis. Further tests such as chest X-ray and a bone scan may be done to see whether the cancer has spread to those sites.

Treatment

In the early stages, when the cancer is confined to the kidney alone, surgery is usually the first treatment, followed by chemotherapy to deal with any tiny cancer cells that may not have been removed, to reduce the risk of relapse. Sometimes chemotherapy may be given before surgery to shrink the tumour and make it easier to operate on. In the later stages, radiotherapy may be used as well.

For children who have advanced disease with metastases, chemotherapy is used as first treatment, sometimes with surgery to remove the metastases afterwards.

Prognosis

The combined approach to treatment, using surgery, radiotherapy, and chemotherapy has led to dramatic improvements in cure rates for Wilm's tumour, from 15 per cent in the 1950s to 90 per cent nowadays. Even children who have widespread metastases have a very good chance of being cured.

Retinoblastoma

This is a cancer of the retina. It is the most common tumour to affect the eye in children, although overall it is very rare, accounting for only 3 per cent of all childhood cancers. About 40 per cent of all cases are caused by an inherited genetic defect. If a parent carries this genetic defect, there is a 50 per cent chance that their child will develop retinoblastoma. This cancer is most common in children under the age of two.

Presentation

The most obvious and common symptom is the 'cat's eye reflex'—the child has a white cast in the pupil of one eye which seems to reflect the light. The other common sign is a squint.

Investigations

A specialist ophthalmologist can usually make a firm diagnosis by looking into the affected eye with an ophthalmoscope. Further tests may include CT or MRI scans and a special kind of ultrasound. Tests will also be done to check for metastases in the central nervous system.

Treatment

Once again, multidisciplinary treatment is the key to the successful treatment of this cancer. The basic treatment used to be, and often still is, the removal of the affected eye by surgery, but advances in radiotherapy have meant that some children no longer need to have this surgery, and the cancer can be treated without their losing their sight in that eye.

If the cancer is diagnosed at an early stage, cryotherapy (freezing the tumour) may be helpful in treating small tumours while radiotherapy can be given for slightly larger tumours, either by external beam, or by means of radioactive discs attached to the back of the eye. Considerable success has been achieved in curing early retinoblastomas in this way. For more advanced disease, chemotherapy may sometimes be used in combination with radiotherapy to try to preserve the eye. In some cases, however, removal of the eye is likely to be necessary. Adjuvant chemotherapy is given to some children after their eye has been removed, to reduce the risks of the cancer returning, and some children also need a course of radiotherapy to the eye socket after removal.

Prognosis

Over 90 per cent of children with retinoblastoma are cured with modern treatments, and many of those children retain their sight in the affected eye. It is vitally important that children with this cancer should be treated in specialist national centres, so that they have the best chance, both of cure and of preserving their sight.

The treatment of children with cancer is one of the great success stories of the last twenty years. Increasingly, now, the attention of health professionals in this field is turning to some of the other issues that arise for these children; for example the long-term effects of intensive cancer treatment at a young age on their growth and development. In addition to the physical effects of such treatment, there are also many psychosocial consequences; for example a child who has spent long periods in hospital may miss out on some of the 'landmark' events of a normal childhood (starting kindergarten or school for example). All specialist children's cancer units have teachers attached to the ward, who maintain links with the child's school and try to ensure that children do not fall behind, and many children return to school quickly after having treatment. In addition, families may find it very difficult dealing with the stress of having a critically ill child, and other children in the family may suffer too. All-round support for the whole family is now increasingly seen as just as vital a part of the care of a child with cancer as first-class medical attention.

9 Quality of life during cancer treatment

●●

One very critical issue for people with cancer, and one that doctors and other health professionals who treat them are increasingly concerned with, is 'quality of life'. Essentially, this means what makes life worth living, but its definition varies from one person to another; what one person may find quite tolerable, for example in terms of side-effects of a treatment, or reduced capability after an operation, another person may find almost unbearable. Nevertheless, many people do readily accept that when they have a disease like cancer (or indeed many other chronic diseases such as arthritis or angina) there has to be some trade-off between quality of life and quantity—that is to say, treatment to prolong life may itself make life more uncomfortable or circumscribed than it used to be. Most people are prepared to put up with a diminution of their 'quality of life' because life itself has value to them.

One study asked people with cancer who were about to have chemotherapy, with known side-effects, what chance of cure they would be prepared to accept. Patients felt that even a 1 per cent chance of cure made the unpleasantness of treatment worthwhile, in contrast to the control group, of people who were not ill, who believed they would only accept the treatment if there was a much higher chance of cure. This study highlighted a number of important issues for health professionals treating people with cancer: that people's attitudes towards treatment and towards their own life and happiness change when they have a life-threatening disease; that people who do not have the disease cannot easily imagine what it is like to be in that situation, and that people who are not ill cannot predict with certainty what someone who is ill would want.

When treatment is given with the realistic hope of curing a cancer, most people accept a temporary reduction in their quality of life, in the expectation that they will get better. Some treatments can be quite toxic (for example very intensive chemotherapy followed by bone marrow or stem cell transplant) and can sometimes make people feel very ill. However, when cure is the priority, most people feel that the discomfort is worthwhile.

Since, at the present time, many cancers are not curable, much treatment is given with the intention of prolonging good quality life. While it is easy to measure the length of someone's life, it is very much harder to measure its quality, since this depends on many different aspects of a person's physical, emotional, mental, and spiritual wellbeing.

Palliative treatments—treatments which are given to alleviate symptoms, shrink and control tumours, and prolong life—often themselves cause side-effects. (These treatments—for example, radiotherapy and chemotherapy—are, after all, the same as those used for curative purposes, though often at lower doses or for shorter periods.) When a doctor is considering such treatment for someone with cancer, then a careful balance has to be drawn between effectiveness and side-effects. If a treatment has few or no side-effects, but does not have much activity against the cancer either, then there is no point in prescribing it at all. The doctor's task is to prescribe the most effective treatment with the fewest possible side-effects.

Cancers can sometimes cause local and specific symptoms, for example if a tumour presses on a nerve it can cause pain, or a tumour can cause a partial blockage or obstruction, e.g. of the airways or the intestine. These symptoms can respond very well to local treatments, such as laser therapy, or radiotherapy to the tumour, to cause it to shrink and thereby relieve the problem. At other times, people with cancer experience more general symptoms, for example, caused by cancers in several parts of the body, or perhaps by some chemical released by the tumour. Such non-specific symptoms might include weight loss, nausea, tiredness, or pain in several parts of the body. While some drugs have been developed specifically to combat some of these symptoms (for example anti-emetics to counteract nausea), often the most effective way of relieving them is to shrink the cancer. Often, shrinking the tumour, even only a little, can afford quite dramatic relief from the symptoms.

Several studies have compared the outcome of treatment with intensive chemotherapy, with more severe side-effects, with a less intensive drug regime with fewer side-effects but correspondingly less activity against the cancer. These studies have shown that quality of life was better after the more intensive treatment, because in the cases studied it was more effective at shrinking the cancer and relieving the symptoms caused by the cancer.

Chemotherapy still has the reputation for being a very unpleasant treatment, causing severe nausea, vomiting and hair loss. When it is suggested as a palliative treatment, patients and their families may be horrified at the thought that such an ordeal is necessary when there is no possibility of cure. In fact, as discussed below and on p.56–62, many recent developments in chemotherapy have been aimed at alleviating or completely avoiding the worst of these side-effects. Nevertheless, because of the history of the development of this treatment, the myths still hold a powerful grasp on the public's imagination.

In the late 1960s and early 1970s, it became apparent that combinations of drugs, many of which were very toxic, could cure certain cancers such as lymphomas and teratomas. Not surprisingly, there was enormous excitement amongst cancer doctors who began to hope that the right combination of drugs would cure most common cancers, and they tried different combinations of drugs in all advanced cancers to find, by trial and error, the right combination for each condition. As a result of this activity during the 1970s, cancer doctors now have a huge amount of information about the drugs: which are active and for which cancers, the most appropriate doses and ways of administering them. From the point of view of scientific research this was an exciting and fruitful period. From the perspective of someone who received those treatments, and experienced many of the side-effects, and from the perspective of his or her relatives, however, this period may seem to have been one of little benefit and much suffering. The situation is much improved nowadays.

Cancer doctors, benefiting from the work of earlier decades now know the drugs extremely well—when they can be useful and at what doses and schedules. Drugs can now be used with maximum effect and minimum side-effects. New generations of the drugs have been developed which are more effective against the cancer and also have fewer side-effects. As doctors and the pharmaceutical industry develop new drugs, the question of lessening side-effects is given a very high priority. Patients who are involved in clinical trials of drugs are often asked to complete 'quality of life' questionnaires. In order to compare a new treatment with one already in standard use, they need to be able to assess the impact of the treatment on patients' own perceptions of their quality of life as well as prolongation of life.

Much better drugs have been developed to counteract side-effects of treatment. This is particularly so in the field of anti-sickness drugs which are now so effective that nausea and vomiting can usually be very well controlled and often not experienced at all.

There are now many different drugs. If one drug does not suit another can be tried, or a different regimen. It is therefore now easier to find ways of making drug treatment tolerable for most people who need it.

Using drugs to treat cancer is a very complex matter. The difference between using drugs well and using them badly may be the difference between the patient having a very difficult time and a reasonable time. Sometimes, even, it can be the difference between life and death. It is therefore very important that anyone with cancer who is going to have chemotherapy should be seen by an oncologist, a doctor who is expert in the use of drug treatments for cancer.

Cancer drugs are expensive. In some cases, some patients may not get the best drug treatment available because of budgetary restrictions in the hospital where they are being treated. People with cancer, or their relatives may have to be assertive with their doctor or hospital to ensure that they do see the appropriate specialist for their kind of illness and treatment, and that the treatment they are getting is the best available.

In the early days of chemotherapy for advanced cancer, both doctors and patients had unrealistic expectations. When these hopes were not fulfilled, many people were disillusioned. It is very important that when palliative treatment is given, doctors are honest about their intentions in giving the treatment, and do not hold out false hopes of a cure. Although not everyone benefits from palliative treatment, many people find that active treatment improves their quality of life and also gives realistic hope, not of cure, but of helping their condition. Hope itself improves their sense of wellbeing and for many people, life without hope may be unbearable. Victor Frankl, in his book *Man's search for meaning*, commented that people in Nazi concentration camps who maintained a hopeful attitude survived longer than those who lost hope, who quickly succumbed to disease.

The effect of complementary therapy and alternative therapy on quality of life

Complementary therapies are usually regarded as those which people use *in addition* to their standard treatment for cancer, while alternative therapies are those which people use *instead* of conventional cancer treatment. Many doctors also regard as alternative treatments those therapies which have been oversold and lead to unrealistic expectations—leading to the same problems of disillusionment and disappointment as did the early use of chemotherapy. Complementary and alternative therapies are discussed in more detail in Chapter 11. Here we look at the contribution they can make to the quality of life of people with cancer.

A number of studies have looked at the use of complementary therapies by people who have cancer. In general, people choose to use these treatments because they hope it might help their cancer, but more importantly because it gives people a feeling that they are doing something positive to help themselves and take control of their lives.

A study done in the United States found that 13 per cent of people receiving cancer treatment also had complementary therapy of some kind, predominantly diets or megavitamins. Studies showed that those who had complementary therapy had a poorer quality of life than people who had conventional treatment alone. In contrast, a survey in the United Kingdom showed that a similar percentage of cancer patients used some form of complementary therapy, but the majority used more psychological approaches such as spiritual healing, visualization, relaxation, or simple physical techniques such as massage and aromatherapy. Most people interviewed in this survey felt that these treatments helped them cope, and that their quality of life had been improved. Though this was not a randomized trial, it nevertheless highlights some interesting features about the kinds of complementary therapies that led to improved quality of life, namely the physical techniques such as massage and the more psychological therapies such as relaxation; the dietary therapies caused significant side-effects including loss of appetite and weight and generally feeling unwell in some patients.

Many cancer treatment centres now offer some forms of complementary therapy, such as relaxation, massage, and aromatherapy, alongside conventional treatment, in the hope that these may improve people's sense of wellbeing, but not in the expectation that they will affect the progress of the cancer in any way. Spiritual healing is the most commonly used complementary therapy in the UK and the decision to seek this form of healing is a very personal one for each individual to take. Few doctors would object to someone with cancer taking this step, and it would not be appropriate for them to object. Most of the disagreements between cancer doctors and complementary practitioners arise in the area of dietary therapies, which most cancer doctors believe to be unhelpful and occasionally positively harmful. Doctors are also alarmed by the sometimes unrealistic hopes that can be raised.

The effect of emotional support, counselling, and psychotherapy on quality of life

Cancer is very frightening. A multitude of powerful and sometimes conflicting emotions can arise; disbelief and denial, anger, grief, guilt, fear, and resentment. People who have cancer also find themselves suddenly locked into a world of unfamiliar and perhaps forbidding hospitals and treatments, their bodies and even their lives suddenly out of their control. Their friends and relatives too will probably experience strong and frightening emotions. Having cancer yourself, or being close to someone who has cancer, can be a time of very great stress which can put huge pressures on relationships, work, and home life. Emotional support is crucially important to people with cancer at every stage of their illness. This can come from many sources. For most people with cancer, the support of their family and friends is invaluable. Many people also find that being given time by their doctors and the nurses looking after them can be very helpful. Cancer is confusing and complex, and many people are frightened of the unknown. Health professionals who can give the time to explain accurately, in detail and with kindness about the illness and the treatments that are being prescribed can be a most powerful source of emotional support.

Many people find that they often feel insecure and anxious if they have been treated in hospital and are then discharged home. Having a telephone number which will put them through to the ward where they were treated, 24 hours a day, so that their queries can be answered by a nurse or one of the junior doctors on duty can be very reassuring.

Telephone helplines and cancer information services, too, such as BACUP in the UK and the Cancer Information Service (CIS) in the US, where qualified professionals can answer questions by telephone or letter, can be enormously supportive. People find these facilities helpful as they can discuss their fears and uncertainties with someone at the other end of the telephone, when they occur, rather than having to wait until they next see their doctor. The anonymity provided by such services may also be helpful. People may have anxieties about which they feel embarrassed to talk face-to-face with their doctor, but which they can feel comfortable discussing over a phone helpline.

For some people, the experience of having cancer creates emotional issues which require more time and expertise than can be provided by family, friends, or doctor. Counselling, either individually or in groups, can be very helpful in allowing people time to discuss their fears and anxieties and to help them cope with the stresses their illness brings. A professional counsellor, preferably one who has some knowledge of cancer, can help people find their way through the tangle of emotions that cancer brings, provide a safe place for people to say some of the things that perhaps they cannot say to anyone close to them, and encourage people to look at some of the fears and uncertainties that are haunting them. Many people find that even a short period of counselling, of perhaps 6 to 8 sessions, leaves them feeling much more in control and able to cope. Group counselling can often be useful to people with cancer, and it offers the opportunity to meet other people in a similar position, who can share their experiences; having cancer can be very lonely, and meeting other people who are in the same boat can be enormously reassuring.

For some people, the emotional problems their cancer brings may require more in-depth therapy, and their doctor can refer them to a psychotherapist, preferably one who specializes in the particular needs of people with cancer.

Conclusion

Many people recover successfully from cancer; many others live for many years with their cancer well controlled. Nevertheless, for most people, the experience of having cancer is profoundly significant and changes their lives in many ways. It can sometimes offer people the opportunity to re-evaluate their lives and to assess and come to understand what is really important to them. Having cancer is a crisis and a challenge, and people can respond to such crises and challenges by finding strengths and abilities within themselves of which they were unaware.

10 *Living with advanced cancer*

Cancers are usually described as advanced if they have spread from the primary site and formed metastases (secondary cancers) in other parts of the body. The reason cancer spreads is that cancer cells break away from the primary tumour and are circulated around the body either in the bloodstream or in the lymphatic system, coming to lodge in other organs or structures of the body; the most common sites for secondary cancers to develop are the lymph glands, the liver, the bones, the lungs, and the brain. As we have explained in the sections on individual cancers, secondary cancers, wherever they are in the body, retain the characteristics of their 'parent' cancer, and respond to the same drug treatment as is effective for the primary. A lung cancer metastasis which is growing in the bones is treated as lung cancer, not as bone cancer.

Some cancers, even when they have spread, are still curable. Others, however, cannot be cured but can be controlled, sometimes for years. So some people who have advanced cancer live for a long time, and may in fact die of something quite unrelated to their cancer; others however may die after a relatively short time. Sometimes doctors do not know whether a particular treatment will prolong life and therefore treatment will be given primarily to improve quality of life, with, as a secondary aim, the hope that some prolongation of life may be achieved.

We have described the treatments for advanced cancers elsewhere in this book, in the sections on the individual cancers. There are, however, a number of other, more general aspects to living with advanced cancer; those we shall consider here are:

- living with the symptoms of cancer

- living with uncertainty

- coping with the possibility of dying.

Living with the symptoms of cancer

Effective pain and symptom control has in the last few decades come to be seen as very important in the care of people with cancer. Cancer itself can cause very distressing symptoms, and the treatments too can cause side-effects which, if not treated, are difficult to tolerate. As treatments to control cancer and prolong life effectively have been developed, so too have doctors developed specialist skills in treating and controlling symptoms so that the benefit gained from the treatment can be life of good quality.

Pain

Perhaps the symptom of cancer that most people anticipate and fear is pain. In fact, many people do not experience much or any pain from their cancer. For those who do, there are now many ways in which pain can be very effectively controlled or even eliminated in almost all patients. It should never be accepted that pain cannot be controlled, and specialist advice should be sought if pain is being experienced and the existing medication is not relieving it adequately. This is an area of medicine in which there have been many advances in recent years, not only in the development of new and better analgesic drugs, but also in other techniques for reducing or stopping pain.

There are many reasons why cancer may cause pain. The tumour may be pressing on a nerve or on the surrounding tissues. Metastases can cause pain in the bones. Inflammation or infection around or near the tumour can be painful, and the site of an operation can also be very sore. Many people fear that pain indicates that their cancer is getting worse. This is not necessarily so. The amount of pain experienced is not in any way linked with the seriousness of the disease.

Another common fear is of becoming addicted to painkillers, and some people put off asking for help for the pain they experience because they fear that they will then embark on an inevitable course of ever stronger drugs in ever increasing doses. In fact, there are now so many different drugs, and the doses can be so finely tuned, that many people remain on mild painkillers for a long time; alternatively, they may be put on a fairly strong painkiller, which may later be reduced when the pain is under control, or if other techniques can be used succesfully in tandem with the drugs. Addiction is extremely rare when strong painkillers are used to treat pain, rather than when they are abused for 'recreational' purposes. No one understands why this is so.

The drugs available range from mild painkillers which can be bought over the counter from a pharmacy (such as aspirin, paracetamol, and ibuprofen), through stronger analgesics such as codeine, dextropropoxyphene, or buprenorphine (which are only available on prescription), to morphine and diamorphine. These drugs may be used in combination so that the pain can be attacked in several ways at once. For example, drugs such as paracetamol, codeine, and morphine often work very effectively with anti-inflammatory drugs such as aspirin and ibuprofen. The painkillers work in the brain and nervous system, where the pain is recorded, while the anti-inflammatory drugs work directly at the site of the pain, reducing swelling and inflammation.

Drugs are most often given orally, either as a tablet or as a liquid. Some may be given as suppositories or as an injection. Morphine can be given in a slow release tablet, which can give continuous pain control for up to about twelve hours, or as an injection. For some people, whose pain is difficult to control, a very effective way of giving morphine is to deliver it via a small pump attached to a syringe, which delivers a continuous drip of the drug under the skin. Diamorphine, or heroin, is very similar to morphine and has a very similar effect but the doses are slightly different.

Most drugs are given every four hours or so. It is important to take the drugs regularly, to prevent the pain, rather than to wait until the pain starts up again. If the dosage prescribed wears off, and the pain comes back before the next dose is due, it is sensible to advise the doctor so that the drugs can be changed or the dosage altered to ensure this does not happen. The aim of pain control is to prevent pain. If the drugs and the dosage are not right, and the patient is experiencing pain, he or she should go back to their doctor to get a more effective regimen.

Some painkillers do cause side-effects. Drowsiness can be a problem, and if affected it is necessary to take care about driving or operating machinery. The doctor should be asked about whether or not alcohol can be drunk while taking these drugs. Constipation is a very common side-effect of painkillers, and many doctors prescribe a laxative at the same time.

Low doses of radiotherapy can be very effective in controlling the source of pain, especially in the bones, but also in other sites, particularly where a tumour is pressing on a nerve or organ. The treatment can cause the tumour to shrink and relieve the pressure; sometimes even quite a small amount of shrinkage can dramatically decrease the amount of pain felt.

Other techniques used by doctors include nerve blocks. By blocking (freezing, heating, or injecting long-acting anaesthetic into) the appropriate nerve, painful messages can be prevented from reaching the brain. Other methods can be used to stimulate the brain to release endorphins, substances the body produces itself as its own painkillers. Such methods include TENS (transcutaneous electrical nerve stimulation), which uses very low electrical currents, and acupuncture. Some people with cancer find these methods very helpful.

Any form of relaxation can also be helpful in relieving pain. Fear and anxiety tend to cause people to tense up, and to intensify discomfort and pain. Anything which helps people to relax and to relieve physical tensions, a relaxation or visualization session, a massage, or just a warm bath and a hot drink, can improve people's spirits and make pain more tolerable. A chance to talk to someone about fears—whether this is a doctor or nurse, a professional counsellor, a religious leader, or just a chat with a friend—can also greatly help to unburden people's minds and therefore relieve physical tensions as well. Doctors may sometimes prescribe a short course of tranquillizers, sleeping pills or anti-depressants if they feel that this will be helpful in relieving anxiety, or if fears, tension, or depression are preventing someone from sleeping.

Eating problems

Many cancers and their side-effects can cause eating and digestive problems, and these can be distressing if they continue, as eating and mealtimes play a very important part in the lives of many people—not just in terms of the pleasure they get from food but also in the part meals play in their social and family relationships. Nausea and vomiting are well known side-effects of chemotherapy, and to a lesser extent radiotherapy, but there are now very effective drugs to prevent and control these distressing symptoms and they are much less of a problem than they used to be. Less well known are other effects such as taste changes, a dry or sore mouth, general loss of appetite, and bowel and bladder problems. All these can have quite profound effects on how people feel about food and mealtimes. If people lose a lot of weight, this can also compromise their general state of health, so it is important to get these problems sorted out, so that he or she can eat as normally as possible.

The doctor will be able to help by prescribing anti-emetics for feelings of sickness and nausea, laxatives for constipation, and medicines for diarrhoea. Sore mouths can be treated with mouthwashes and sometimes anaesthetic ointment or gel, and the patient will probably also be taught the elements of mouthcare in order to lessen the risk of this happening. If weight loss occurs a short course of a progesterone, such as medroxyprogesterone acetate, or megestrol may be prescribed, to help put some weight back on. In addition, it may be helpful to speak to a dietician who may be able to give useful information and hints about diet and how best to prepare foods so that they are both nutritious and tempting. The dietician will also be able to give advice about the various nutritious drinks and dietary supplements available (which may be available on prescription). These can be used to replace meals and contain all the nutrients needed in an easily digestible form. A very helpful booklet is obtainable from BACUP (see Appendix). Entitled *Diet and the cancer patient*, it provides a lot of information about eating problems commonly experienced and suggests ways of coping with them.

Breathing problems

Sometimes cancer, or its side-effects can cause people to have difficulty in breathing, perhaps wheezing, or coughing, or feeling short of breath. Radiotherapy to the chest can cause breathlessness too. The doctor will investigate the cause of these symptoms, and there are many ways in which they can be relieved. If they are caused by infection, antibiotics can be given to clear it up. If the airways in the lungs have gone into spasm (similar to an asthma attack), drugs can help to widen the airways and make breathing easier. If fluid has built up around the lungs it can be removed; the doctor can draw it off through a syringe, under a local anaesthetic, or, if the problem persists, a small drainage tube can be inserted into the chest and the liquid drawn off as necessary. Following the drainage, the doctor may inject a substance into the chest to prevent a recurrence of the fluid.

Lymphoedema and ascites

Lymphoedema is a swelling up of an arm or leg, caused by a build up of fluid in the limb. This usually happens because the lymph glands have either been affected by the cancer, or have been removed at an operation to check for spread of the cancer. It is most common in women who have had surgery for breast cancer and occurs much less commonly in people who have lymphomas. More rarely it can occur with other cancers. Removal of the lymph glands interferes with the normal process by which lymphatic fluid drains from the limb, and it therefore builds up and causes swelling. This can be exacerbated by subsequent radiotherapy. The affected arm or leg can be painful, heavy and awkward to use and people often find it embarrassing too, as it can be a very visible sign of their illness.

Many hospitals now run lymphoedema clinics especially to help with the management of this condition. Treatment usually involves massage, to drain the fluid away from the limb, and also the use of special bandages to control and prevent the swelling. It is important to look after the skin on the swollen arm or leg very carefully as it can easily become broken and infected.

Some cancers can cause fluid to build up in the abdomen, causing it to swell up and become uncomfortable. This is called ascites. The fluid can be drained off in a very simple procedure under local anaesthetic.

Sweats and itching

Some cancers can cause sudden profound sweating, and others can cause itchiness of the skin. Drugs may be prescribed to control these symptoms. Meanwhile, wearing light clothing, preferably made of natural fibres like cotton and wool can be helpful; care that any products used on the skin (such as soap, lotions, talc etc.) are not causing further irritation, and perhaps changing the brand to a gentle unperfumed kind are all things worth trying. Washing powders too can cause skin to become irritated. At night, the bedroom should not be too hot, and the bedclothes should be light.

No one will have all of these problems and many people will have none of them. With all these symptoms, the most important thing to do is to tell the doctor about them as soon as they start to be troublesome. There are many ways in which people can be helped and the symptoms prevented and there are many very experienced and specialist health professionals working in this field whose expertise can be called on if needed.

Living with uncertainty

Many people say that this is one of the hardest things about living with cancer. It can be very frustrating and saddening to find that hopes and plans for the future have been overturned by illness. Even very short-term plans may be difficult to make if the person is not sure from one day to the next whether they will feel fit enough to carry them out.

It is natural for someone with cancer to have many fears and anxieties about the progress of their illness, and at times these fears may seem to dominate their thoughts for every waking moment. But these burdens do not have to be shouldered alone. There are many sources of support, help, and information, and these can be invaluable in helping people to cope with their fears. Often people find that when they have had the opportunity to address their fears, they feel that they can then set them aside, and concentrate on living in the here and now.

One of the most important sources of information is the cancer doctor. Although no doctor can ever predict exactly what will happen in anyone's individual case, she or he will have the experience to be able to answer questions about the likely progress of the illness and what treatments are available at every stage. The patient should not feel hesitant or embarrassed to ask their doctor about anything they feel they need to know.

If there is something they are determined to do, for example, to make a trip somewhere or attend an important event such as a family wedding, it is valuable to enlist the doctor's support as soon as possible. He or she may be able to help by, for example, rescheduling treatment, or temporarily altering the drug dosage or regimen, to ensure that the patient is feeling their best and can achieve what they have set their heart on.

The family doctor may also play an important role, especially for the patient at home. He or she will know of the local availability of help and support; for example a cancer support group, or the facilities of a local hospice, or the availability of specially trained nurses who can visit the home.

Practical concerns can be very worrying at this time. These may be financial or work-related problems, or anxieties about no longer being able to get about easily or to care for oneself. Once again, it is better not to let these things weigh on the mind, but to seek help as soon as the problems arise. The bank manager, mortgage lender, solicitor, financial adviser or workplace welfare officer may need to be contacted and informed of the illness. A social worker, contacted through the hospital involved in the care, or the doctor or nurse can identify the benefits which the patient may be entitled to claim, and can also arrange for care at home—for example by arranging help in the house, or special equipment to help maintain independence.

Living with the uncertainty that cancer brings is very stressful, both for the person who is ill and for his or her relatives and friends. The emotional temperature can become very high, as everyone struggles with powerful and sometimes overwhelming feelings. Many people find it helpful to talk to someone who is outside their immediate circle, to vent some of the pent-up emotions, and perhaps try and sort out in their own mind some of the problems which may be making their relationships and friendships fraught at a time when they most need to be strong and supportive. The sympathetic ear of a friend, a talk with a nurse, social worker, minister, rabbi, or other religious leader, may be all that is needed, but sometimes more formal counselling either alone or in a group can be more rewarding (see p.222–223 for more about counselling).

Many people find it very saddening and frustrating to have to let go of the life they used to lead and adapt to the physical constraints of their illness. For example, someone who has always been the nurturer and carer of a family may find it very difficult to accept caring and nursing from others. Or the family's wage earner may feel their role has been diminished because they can no longer go out to work. On the other hand, many people have, perhaps paradoxically, welcomed the opportunity their illness has provided to sort out their priorities and concentrate on the things they enjoy. They speak of a heightened appreciation of sights and sounds, and a greater satisfaction in small pleasures than perhaps their busy lives had allowed them time for before they became ill.

I feel almost guilty saying this, but cancer can have a good side too.

I've never been so generally happy as I am now. Some moments in nature, and my general feeling of loving life are somehow much more important now. The colours are more intense, everything is more beautiful and I wouldn't miss it for anything in the world. The strange thing is that I never noticed so many things before I was diagnosed as having cancer.

A woman with cancer, quoted in *Challenging cancer: from chaos to control* by Nira Kfir and Maurice Slevin, Tavistock/Routledge 1991.

Coping with the possibility of dying

Once again, it must be emphasized that some cancers, even when advanced, can be cured, and other advanced cancers can be controlled for many years. Nevertheless, there may come a time when it becomes apparent that recovery is not going to occur. Some people indeed, decide themselves that they do not want further active treatment. People often report that someone with cancer has been told by doctors 'there is nothing more we can do for you'. No responsible doctor should ever say that. It may be that curative treatments are no longer working, but there are always palliative measures and support and care that can be given to make people's remaining life as comfortable, independent, and dignified as possible. Doctors do not wash their hands of patients if they cannot cure them, and indeed the care of people who are terminally ill with cancer has in recent years become one of increasing activity and interest.

Many people want their doctor to estimate how long they have got to live. Doctors cannot give a definite answer, not because they are ducking an awkward question, but because statistical figures, derived from studies of large numbers of people with cancer, cannot be applied in an individual case, as the progress of every cancer varies widely. Some doctors may give a rough estimate, but would probably hedge it with caveats. An over-optimistic prediction risks the person who is ill perhaps postponing decisions or procrastinating about dealing with important issues, and may result in bitter disappointment if the illness worsens unexpectedly; on the other hand a pessimistic prediction is equally unhelpful. It is often most accurate to give a range of possible life expectancy, but to emphasize that even a very broad range may be wrong.

It is very common and natural for people to worry about how they will be looked after as their illness progresses. Some people want to be at home, and there are many agencies who can help to make this possible; the cancer doctor, family doctor, and/or social worker can explain what is available. Other people feel more secure being cared for by health professionals in a hospital or hospice.

The hospice movement has been in the forefront of the development of better ways of looking after people who are terminally ill, especially people with cancer. The emphasis in hospice care is on controlling symptoms, improving quality of life, and providing care and support to enable people to die with dignity. Hospices tend to be calm and, perhaps surprisingly, cheerful places, where the pace is less rushed than in a normal hospital. Relatives and even sometimes family pets are welcomed, and support to the family of the person who is ill is seen as an integral part of the care the hospice gives.

People do not only go into hospices when they are dying. They may sometimes go in for a short period, for example to have their symptoms monitored and brought under control, before going home again. In addition some hospices run day centres, and many have teams of nurse specialists (home care teams) who can visit people living at home and offer advice on pain and symptom control.

One strategy that many people adopt when faced with the knowledge that their life is limited is to prepare for the worst and live for the best. Putting their affairs in order—for example, making a will, listing the whereabouts of important documents, or addresses of important people, writing letters, even sometimes planning their funeral—can sometimes provide a way in which people can come to terms with the idea of their own death. Many people at this time like to go over their own life, perhaps looking at old photographs, or just reflecting. Sometimes they may want to get in touch with old friends, or deal with 'unfinished business' such as old hurts or emotional loose ends. Then, with the practical affairs dealt with, many people feel more free to concentrate on living each day as it comes and working towards the best possible outcome.

Coming to terms with the idea of dying is never easy. People who are dying often go through the same stages of grieving as do people who have been bereaved. Here again, psychological and emotional support, whether from friends and relatives, nursing and medical staff, a counsellor, a support group, or a religious leader, can be invaluable in helping people through this painful and difficult process.

11 Complementary medicine in cancer care by Dr Tim Sheard

This chapter is presented as a brief and simple review of the complementary therapies commonly used by people with cancer. It is intended for reference and in order to make the information easily accessible each therapy is described under the following headings.

What it is, possible benefits, common problems/dangers, and availability

This logical approach should make the chapter easy to use. However, it is done at the expense of conveying or emphasizing the crucial subjective, emotional, intuitive, and poetic aspects of complementary medicine. This can be remedied by reading other books and, more importantly, by direct experience of complementary therapies.

Before starting it is important to look at what we mean by 'the facts'. This is a controversial area and the person approaching it for the first time may be surprised at the contradictory 'facts' to be found in different books or articles. One reason for this is that many authors fail to distinguish between opinions, common sense views, and reliable established facts. Another reason is that different authors are viewing cancer care from very different perspectives. Medicine has only been able to advance so much and so rapidly in this last century because of the use of scientific research to distinguish facts from impressions, opinions, fashions, or prejudices. An historical example of the importance of scientific research is the abandonment of the routine use of radical mastectomy to treat breast cancer (this was an operation in which the whole breast, underlying muscles, and lymph glands in the armpit were removed. See p.94). Research showed conclusively that, in most cases, other simpler, less mutilating operations with fewer side-effects were just as effective in treating the cancer.

Sadly we do not yet have the benefit of research facts on complementary therapies in cancer care. What we must base decisions on in the meantime is informed opinion, founded on and tempered by experience, while trying to avoid sheer prejudice based on ignorance.

It is the intention of this chapter to present an informed opinion; however, it is recommended that the interested reader look at other books, many written from a non-medical viewpoint, which offer different and sometimes contradictory perspectives.

Complementary medicine in cancer care

What it is

It is not clear where exactly to draw the line between complementary and conventional medicine and nursing care. For the purposes of this chapter complementary medicine is taken as that which is not normally available for those who are being treated for cancer in normal hospital wards but which is intended to be used alongside normal medical and nursing care. This is different from 'alternative medicine' which is often presented as a substitute for conventional medicine.

Complementary means 'serving to complete'. The ways in which complementary therapies can be understood to be serving to complete modern, technological cancer medicine are in:

- focusing on helping the *person* with cancer (and partners, relatives, and supporters) rather than treatment of the *disease* cancer itself

- trying to approach the whole person, the mind, body, social relationships, and spirit

- seeking to heal, or 'make whole' the person as distinct from curing the disease

- helping people to actively help themselves; this contrasts with the tendency for people to become passive and dependent when receiving medical treatment.

Possible benefits

- To help people with cancer to find their own way of dealing with and/or finding their own meaning in the situation. This may help them to adjust more positively to having cancer, the threat of recurrence, or the process of dying.

- To help regain some sense of control or influence through active participation.
- To help to positively involve relatives and friends.
- To help with symptom control.
- Overall to help with quality of life.

Common problems and dangers
- It is possible to confuse a sense of control in life with control over the actual disease itself. This can lead to using complementary therapies as a treatment for cancer itself: there is as yet no scientific or reliable evidence that complementary therapies make any difference to how long people with cancer live. Some people claim otherwise and base their opinion upon individual case histories or remarkable recoveries.

- Some people set up complementary therapies in opposition or competition with normal medical treatment. It is suggested that complementary therapies are 'good', 'gentle', and 'natural' and that normal medical treatment is some kind of 'warfare on the body'. This kind of very narrow black and white perspective can put people off having beneficial medical treatment and create unnecessary conflict.

- Finally it is quite often put around in the complementary or alternative fields that developing a serious illness like cancer is somehow the individual's own responsibility. People therefore get the idea that it is their 'fault' that they have developed cancer and consequently that they should have control over its progress. This is a grossly simplistic viewpoint on what is a very complex situation. At first this is often stated positively in suggesting that people can reverse the process of the growth of cancer and get rid of it. However such an approach can often cause, or increase a person's sense of guilt or failure in developing cancer or its subsequent progression. An approach which encourages people to become heroes can easily lead to a punishing attitude and feeling of self betrayal.

It can be seen from this that complementary medicine can help to make medicine more holistic: that it is to address the whole person and to help that person become more autonomous, to grow and mature. This holds great promise in helping people with cancer and their supporters, but it is not without side-effects.

Availability

Complementary therapies are increasingly available in hospices and specialist cancer treatment wards in hospitals. Many support groups offer complementary therapies as do some independent centres. Finally there is a fast growing complementary medicine industry in this country supplied by private practitioners who charge fees.

Individual therapies

A limited number of therapies are described. Others, such as reflexology, acupuncture, art therapy, yoga, t'ai chi, homeopathy, cranial osteopathy, and herbalism could have been described in a longer chapter.

Counselling

What it is

Counselling is offering people with cancer and their supporters the opportunity to talk to a professional person in confidence about their thoughts and feelings. This is part of the work of all nurses and doctors involved in cancer care but sometimes people need a specially trained counsellor who has more time, experience, and expertise.

Possible benefits

Having cancer diagnosed may throw people into a crisis by stirring up complex and often overwhelming thoughts and feelings. For most having cancer is an event which has never occurred before in their lives and is very threatening and disturbing. Counselling may help individuals to adjust positively to this change by helping to:

- support them in facing the diagnosis and its implications

- openly express and explore (perhaps conflicting) thoughts and feelings about it
- formulate a way forward
- facilitate adjustments, changes, and communication within important relationships (such as marriage)
- alleviate tension, anxiety, and depression
- grow through the crisis of cancer, perhaps finding opportunities for enhancement or enrichment of aspects of life
- complete unfinished business and let go.

Common problems and dangers

- There is a common belief that there is a 'cancer personality' that makes some people more prone to developing cancer. Quite a lot of research has been done to try and show a connection between personality and attitude and the development of cancer. So far it has failed to prove it. The idea of a cancer personality is a dangerous and false over-simplification.

- It is also commonly thought that how people react to having cancer will determine or greatly affect whether they will be cured or how long they will live. It is suggested that having a 'fighting spirit' or 'being positive' is good and feeling hopeless or negative is bad and will shorten the person's life. This again is unproven. Research done in London is often quoted as proving that attitude does effect survival. However this is not the case. That particular study had important weaknesses and attempts to repeat it have had mixed and contradictory results.

- Many people think that it has been proven that stress, or stressful events cause cancer and make it progress more rapidly. Again this is not proven although very widely believed among the public.

Availability

In support groups, in hospitals and hospices, through BACUP (see Appendix), private counsellors, psychiatrists, and psychologists. **Beware**: Anyone can call themselves a counsellor with only the most minimum of training. It is important to check a counsellor's qualifications, experience, and professional accreditation.

Relaxation

What it is

Teaching people how to relax their bodies in a 10–20 minute exercise. This can be done through personal instruction either individually or in a group and/or using an audio tape.

Possible benefits

• Helping people to feel good in mind and body.

• Releasing tiring and unpleasant physical tension and anxiety caused by mental or emotional distress.

• Helping release pent up emotions.

• Helping with pain or other symptoms (e.g. nausea and vomiting).

• Helping with sleeplessness.

• Learning to let go and be at peace in stressful circumstances.

Common problems and dangers

Many people say 'I can't relax'. The vast majority of people, with help, can learn to relax.

• Relaxation can release unexpressed feelings like grief or sadness which have been held in, resulting in physical tensions. Such a 'letting go' is very likely to be helpful although it might be distressing at the time.

Availability

Relaxation is widely available through support groups, general practices, hospital, local groups, courses, and through audio tapes sold on the open market.

Visualization

What it is

It is not possible to describe visualization at all adequately in a few sentences. If the reader is interested I suggest trying it out, preferably with experienced help. Superficially it can be seen as using the imagination, through any of the five senses, to help achieve goals.

An example of this in everyday life is visualizing a cake before it is decorated or planning a route in one's mind. It is often used in sport to improve performance. On another level it is the use of the imagination to find different ways of looking at things (e.g. having cancer) in order to gain a different or deeper understanding of life situations or problems. It can therefore help people to find their own unique meaning in, and understanding of, their situation. Using visualization in this way is the opposite of being goal-orientated. It requires a letting go and allowing of spontaneous images or sensations.

Possible benefits

- As an aid to relaxation, meditation, and control of symptoms (e.g. nausea or pain).

- As a way of discovering soothing, restorative, or healing images of the body.

- As a tool in a search for meaning and wholeness.

Common problems and dangers

Some people use visualization as a kind of self hypnosis to try and cure or slow down the growth of the cancer. This is done using images of the cancer being overwhelmed and destroyed by all-powerful forces. I have met people whose confidence seems to have been helped by this type of fighting image but they have been a small minority. This kind of approach can cause problems in setting up a struggle which may result in 'failure' which can then lead to guilt. Another problem is that visualization can be used to build up an excessive denial of the seriousness of the condition.

Availability

Books and audio tapes are available. However anyone wishing to do much visualization is advised to seek help and guidance from a counsellor, support group, relaxation therapist, or healer.

Massage

What it is

Massage needs no introduction except to mention that there are different types:

- Swedish massage which is vigorous and used for fit people, e.g. athletes.

- Holistic/intuitive. This is a gentler and subtler approach.

- Aromatherapy. This is similar to holistic massage but also involves the use of essential oils which have aromatic scents (e.g. lavender, sage, rose).

Possible benefits

- Relaxation, letting go.

- Comfort, human touch, and empathy. A way of expressing and receiving care and love.

- For a debilitated person with an unwell body it can be a particularly welcome pleasurable physical experience.

- Reassurance and acceptance especially for those with sick or damaged bodies.

- Can be done by, and to, both individuals with cancer and their relatives.

Common problems and dangers

Within 48 hours after sustained massage people can experience reactions such as feeling off colour or having odd mild symptoms. This usually leads on to a feeling of benefit and improvement, for example in overall relaxation, release of emotions, and a feeling of wellbeing.

Aromatherapists warn against using certain essential oils on sick people or when they are receiving strong treatment such as chemotherapy or radiotherapy.

Vigorous massage, such as Swedish massage, is not appropriate to someone who is physically debilitated.

Some massage practitioners are wary of massaging people with cancer in case it might actually spread the cancer. This is very unlikely to be a problem, although of course direct massage of actual tumours which can be felt near the surface of the body (e.g. in the breast or armpit) is to be avoided. If in doubt ask your doctor.

Availability

Many nurses in hospices and hospitals have learned some massage techniques. Support groups may also offer it and massage practitioners may be found through making local enquiries. It is important to make sure that they are suitably qualified, and have at least an ITEC or AMP qualification.

Meditation

What it is

Meditation is a calming and focusing of the mind using simple techniques such as concentrating on the breath, repeating words, or looking at a candle flame.

Possible benefits

As in relaxation and healing it is a way of achieving a sense of inner stillness, peace, or perhaps a different perspective on problems and dilemmas. It can also be helpful in symptom control, for example, relief of pain.

Common problems and dangers

Some people, probably a large minority, find it very difficult to do. To achieve stillness involves a balance between concentration and letting go. This requires practice, commitment, and guidance.

Availability

Support groups and churches may offer teaching of meditation. Tapes are available and it is sometimes taught in adult education classes.

Healing or laying on of hands

What it is

Healing is an ancient practice which occurs in many cultures through-out the world. In it the healer may touch the person receiving the healing or hold his or her hand a short distance from the body. To receive healing requires faith only on the part of the healer, not the person seeking healing.

Possible benefits

While receiving healing people sometimes feel strong sensations or emotions. Most however feel some sense of relaxation, peace, or stillness. People claim to have experienced physical, emotional, mental, or spiritual benefit from healing. Attempts have been made to research this and results are so far inconclusive. The most consistent feedback is of people experiencing a sense of renewal, or of help in letting go and finding inner peace. Some have said 'nothing has changed, the cancer hasn't gone away but somehow I feel different and more at peace in myself'.

Common problems/dangers

Sometimes people pin a lot of hope on healing achieving a miracle cure. Cancers do, very occasionally, disappear without medical treatment. This is called spontaneous remission, but it is very, very rare. Clearly somebody approaching healing with this as their main hope is likely to feel disappointed or let down.

Some people do not consider healing an option because their religious viewpoint disagrees with it.

Availability

There are many healers in this country and they are best contacted through the big national organizations who have published codes of conduct. Many healers give their services free of charge, or have a collection box (a small minority do charge fixed fees). Many will also visit ill people in their own homes or in hospital. The national organizations will supply addresses of local contacts.

Dietary change

What it is

This has become an important subject, not I think because of great benefits but rather because it has caused a lot of problems. There have been a number of special diets proposed for the treatment of cancer, e.g. the Gerson diet and naturopathic diet, and others to promote wellbeing.

Possible benefits

There is no reliable evidence that dietary change can cure cancer or affect its progress. There is strong circumstantial evidence that certain dietary factors are important in *causing* cancer but this is a far cry from using diet to treat cancer. Removing possible cancer causing substances from the diet is unlikely to change the situation once cancer has developed. (It would be like trying to cure established lung cancer by giving up smoking.)

On a more positive note, for a number of people it appears that a change in diet has promoted a greater sense of physical wellbeing and energy. It is a very direct form of self help and gives an opportunity for relatives and supporters to be positively involved.

Common problems and dangers

Food is an important part of people's quality of life and sense of cultural identity. It is particularly important in a disease like cancer where appetite and weight loss can be symptoms. Radical dietary change or restriction is therefore potentially dangerous both in terms of physical health and quality of life. A number of people have suffered greatly through dietary change. Anyone contemplating radical change must, at the very least, seek medical advice and support.

Availability

There are many books on the subject and advice can be sought from a good dietitian.

Support groups

What they are

A cancer support group is a regular meeting of individuals with cancer and often their supporters which usually has one or two lay people and/or professionals facilitating it.

Possible benefits

Such a meeting provides mutual support and understanding from those in a similar predicament. It is possible to learn how others have managed certain situations, sharing successes as well as disappointments. People with cancer can often feel very isolated by their illness and meeting others in the same predicament can be extremely helpful.

Common problems and dangers

People often imagine that such a group will be depressing, particularly so when group members die. This is not usually the case, many people are very impressed at the level of humour and the positive outlook such groups have. However if badly led such groups can go wrong in terms of formation of cliques, scapegoating people, or imposing a group culture on each individual member (for example that everyone must 'fight' their cancer). It is worth checking on how long the group has been going and the qualifications and experience of those leading it.

Conclusion

This short chapter has been presented in a factual way to enable readers to have easy access to information. In doing this the crucial subjective, emotional, and poetic aspects of complementary medicine have been largely left out. For the reader who wishes to experience these and to explore complementary therapies further I do recommend direct experience alongside further reading.

Useful addresses

United Kingdom
BACUP
3 Bath Place
Rivington Street
London EC2A 3JR
Freeline: 0800 181199
Tel: 0171 613 2121

Breast Cancer Care
210 New Kings Road
London SW6 4NZ
Tel: 0171 384 2984

British Association of Counselling
1 Regent Place
Rugby CV21 2PJ
Tel: 01788 578328

British Colostomy Association
15 Station Road
Reading
Berks RG1 1LG
Tel: 01734 391537

Cancer Care Society
21 Zetland Road
Redland
Bristol BS6 7AH
Tel: 01272 427419

Cancer Help Centre
Grove House
Cornwallis Grove
Clifton Bristol BS8 4PG
Tel: 01272 743216

CancerLink
17 Britannia Street
London WC1X 9JN
Tel helpline: 0171 833 2451

Cancer & Leukaemia in Childhood
CLIC House
Fremantle Square
Bristol BS6 5T
Tel: 01272 244333

Cancer Relief Macmillan Fund
Anchor House
15/19 Britten Street
London SW3 3TZ
Tel: 0171 351 7811

Cancer Research Campaign
6–10 Cambridge Terrace
Regents Park
London NW1 4JL
Tel: 0171 224 1333

Carers National Assoc.
20–25 Glasshouse Yard
London EC1A 4JS
Tel: 0171 490 8898

The Compassionate Friends
53 North Street
Bristol BS3 1EN
Tel: 01272 539639

Cruse
Bereavement Care
126 Sheen Road
Richmond TW9 1UR
Tel: 0181 940 4818

Hodgkin's Disease Assoc
PO Box 275
Haddenham
Aylesbury Bucks
HP17 8JJ
Tel: 01844 291500

Hospice Information Service
St Christopher's Hospice
51–59 Lawrie Park Road
Sydenham SE26 6DZ
Tel: 0181 778 9252

Hysterectomy Support Network
3 Lynne Close
Green Street Green
Orpington Kent
BR6 6BS

Imperial Cancer Research Fund
PO Box 123
Lincoln's Inn Fields
London WC2A 3PX
Tel: 0171 242 0200

The Leukaemia Care Society
14 Kingfisher Court
Venny Bridge
Pinhoe Devon
EX4 8JN
Tel: 01392 464848

The Malcolm Sargent Cancer
  Fund for Children
14 Abingdon Road
London W8 6AF
Tel: 0171 937 4548

Marie Curie Cancer Care
28 Belgrave Square
London SW1X 8QG
Tel: 0171 235 3325

Mind Over Matter
(Testicular Cancer)
14 Blighmont Crescent
Millbrook
Southampton Hants
SO15 8RH
Answerphone: 0703 775611

National Association of
  Laryngectomee Clubs
Ground Floor
6 Rickett Street
Fulham SW6 1RU
Tel: 0171 381 9993

National Cancer Alliance
PO Box 579
Oxford OX4 1LP
Tel: 01865 793566

The Neuroblastoma Society
41 Towncourt Crescent
Petts Wood Kent
BR5 1PH
Tel: 01689 873338

Oesophageal Patients Association
16 Whitefields Crescent
Solihull
West Midlands B91 3NU
Tel: 0121 704 9860

Retinoblastoma Society
c/o Academic Department of Paediatric
Oncology
St Bartholomew's Hospital
West Smithfield EC1A 7BE
Tel: 0171 600 3309

Save Our Sons
Tides Reach
1 Kite Hill
Wooton Bridge
Isle of Wight PO33 4LA
Tel: evenings 01983 882876

The Sue Ryder Foundation
Cavendish
Sudbury Suffolk
CO10 8AY
Tel: 01787 280252

Urostomy Association
Buckland
Beaumont Park
Danbury
Essex CM3 4DE
Tel: 01245 224294

Womens Nationwide Cancer
Control Campaign
128/130 Curtain Road
London EC2A 3AR
Tel: 0171 729 4688

Tak Tent Cancer Support
The Western Infirmary Block
20 Western Court
100 University Place
Glasgow G12 6SQ
Tel: 0141 211 1930

Tenovus Cancer Information Centre
142 Whitchurch Road
Cardiff CF4 3NA
Tel: 01222 619846

The Ulster Cancer Foundation
40–42 Eglantine Avenue
Belfast BT9 6DX
Tel: 01232 663281

Eire

The Irish Cancer Society
5 Northumberland Road
Dublin 4
Tel: 001 668 1855

**Members of the European Cancer
Leagues in Europe**

Dr Anna Achilleoudi
President
Cyprus Assoc. of Cancer Patients
    and Friends
PO Box 3868, Nicosia
Cyprus

Nicolas Dontas
Hellenic Cancer Society
Pindarou Street 25
Kolonaki
GR-10680
Greece

Nicolas Kordiolis
11 Valtetsiou St
10680 Athens
Greece

Maria Mendez-Nunez
Asociacion Espanola contra
    el Cancer
Amador de los Rios 5
E 28010 Madrid
Spain

Katalin Vasvary
Secretary General
Hungarian Cancer League
Post Box 7
H-1507 Budapest
Hungary

Bob Verburg
Assoc. of Comprehensive
    Cancer Centres
PO Box 19001
3501 DA Utrecht
Holland

Marie-Paule Prost
Ligue Luxembourgeoise
    contre le Cancer
C/O Croix Rouge Luxembourg
L-2014 Luxembourg

Damir Eljuga
Croatian League Against Cancer
Illica 197
CRO-4100 Zagreb
Croatia

Prof Giovanni D'Errico
Lega Italiane per la lotta
Contro I Tumori
Via A Torlonia 15
000-00161 Roma, Italy

Gudrun Agnarsdottir
Krabbameinsfelag Islands
Skogarhlid 8
PO Box 5420
IS 125 Reykjavik
Iceland

Achim Ebert
Deutsche Krebshilfe
Thomas Mann Strasse 40
Postfach 1467
D 5300 Bonn, Germany

Klaas van de Poll &
Monda Heshusius
The Dutch Cancer Society
Sophialaan 8
1075 BR Amsterdam
Holland

Bo Oscarsson
Gencralsekretaer
Cancerfonden
20155 Stockholm
Sweden

Maria Bugeja
Maria Bugeja Cancer
    Support Foundation
55 St Joseph Str.,
Pieta
Malta

Didier van der Steichel
Oeuvre Belge due Cancer
217 rue Royale
B-1210 Bruxelles
Belgium

Francesco Schittulli
Leag Italiana per la lotta
control I tumori
Corso Benedetto Croce 32
I 70125 Bari
Italy

Liisa Elovainio
Cancer Soc. of Finland
Liisankatu 21 B
SF 00170 Helsinki 17
Finland

Mrs Ninna Wursten
Danish Cancer Society
Strandboulcvarden 49
2100 Kobenhavn O
Denmark

Lilly Christensen
Generalsekretaer
Den Norske Kreftforening
Postbox 5327, Majorstua
N-0304 Oslo 3
Norway

Liisa Elovainio
Generalsekretaer
Cancerforeningen i Finland
Liisankatu 21B
SF 00170 Helskinki 17
Finland

Tom Hudson
Chief Executive
The Irish Cancer Society
5 Northumberland Road
Dublin 4
Ireland

Gabriel Pallez
Ligue Nationale Francaise
   contre le Cancer
1 Avenue Stephen Pichon
F-75013 Paris
France

Dr Eva Siracka
President
League Against Cancer
Spitalska 21
SLO-812 32 Bratislava
Slovakia

Maire Sepp
Estonian Cancer Society
Hiiu 44
EE-0107 Tallinn
Estonia

Sabine von Kliest
Inst. fur Immunbiologie
   de Universitat
Stefan-Meier-Strabe 8
D79104 Freiburg
Germany

Jeanne Froideveaux
Swiss Cancer League
Monbijoustrasse 61
CH 3001 Bern
Switzerland

USA

The Cancer Information Service (CIS) is a nationwide network of 19 regional offices supported by the National Cancer Institute (NCI), the U.S. Government's primary agency for cancer research. As the voice of the National Cancer Institute, the CIS serves the public through two programs: a toll-free telephone service and an outreach program. Through its toll-free phone service, the CIS provides accurate, up-to-date information on cancer to patients and their families, health professionals, and the general public.

What kinds of information does the CIS telephone service provide?

The CIS can provide unbiased information in understandable language about specific types of cancer, as well as information on state-of-the-art care and the availability of clinical trials. Each CIS office has access to the National Cancer Institute's *PDO* database, which contains current treatment, early detection, and supportive care information. In addition, the CIS can provide referrals to cancer-related community resources such as FDA-certified mammography facilities. The CIS also distributes to callers *materials* from the National Cancer Institute.

Who answers callers' questions?

Certified Information Specialists trained by the National Cancer Institute use a variety of printed and computerized resources to respond to questions. Although CIS Information Specialists are not doctors, they can provide the most accurate and up-to-date information available from the National Cancer Institute.

How can you reach the Cancer Information Service?

The Cancer Information Service (CIS) can be reached anywhere in the United States and Puerto Rico by dialing: 1-800-4-CANCER (1-800-422-6237) or 1-800-332-8615 TTY. Hours of operation are Monday through Friday, 9:00 a.m. to 4:30 p.m., local time.

Callers are automatically routed to the office that serves their region. The CIS also provides direct TTY service to callers who are hearing impaired. Persons with TTY equipment may call 1-800-332-8615 for cancer information.

You can also E-mail your questions to: icic@aspensys.com

Index

....

adenocarcinoma 85
adrenal gland 143–5, 146
advanced cancer 209–18
    palliation 45–6, 49, 202, 204
aflatoxins 140
airways, obstruction 28–9
alpha-fetoprotein 21, 35, 156
alveolar cell carcinoma 88
aminoglutethimide 98
anti-emetics 213
arteriogram 37
asbestos 87
ascites 101, 141, 214
astrocytomas 78–82
atomic explosion 18

barium enema 36–7
barium swallow 117, 122–3
basal cell carcinoma of skin 167–72
3,4 benzpyrene 4
beta-HGC 35, 156
bile duct obstruction 141
biopsy 44
    cone 109
    excision 93
    needle 93
bladder 42, 149–51
    radiotherapy 54–5
bleeding 32
    bowel 32
    lung 32
blood count 35
blood vessels, obstruction 28–9
bone cancer 160–4
bone marrow
    growth factors 63
    HLA matching 64
    side effects of chemotherapy 60

bone marrow transplantation
    autologous transplants 63
    blood transfusions 65–6
    chemotherapy 65
    collection from patient or donor 64
    graft-versus-host disease 67
    harvest of stem cells 62
    Hodgkin's disease 67
    initial treatment 64
    leukaemias 191
    non-Hodgkin's lymphomas 67
    platelet transfusions 65–6
    purging 64
    risks of infections 65–7
    stem cells 62–8
    total body irradiation 65
bowel 126–34
    bacteria 30–1
    colonoscopy 42
    faecal occult blood tests 25, 128
    inflammatory disease 127
    obstruction 28–9
brain tumours 78–82
breast cancer 23, 88–100
    male 100
    Paget's disease 99–100
    surgery 94–5, 99
breast screening 92–4
    self examination 91
breathing problems 213
bronchoalveolar carcinoma 88
bronchoscopy 41
Burkitt's lymphoma 180

CA-125 101
caesium implants 55
cancer, carcinoma, terminology 1, 7
'cancer personality' 223

carcinogens 4, 87, 149
carcinoid tumours 88, 139
cells
    biology 2–4
    DNA 2–4
    mutations 4
cervix 24, 105–12
    CIN (cervical intraepithelial neoplasia)
        106
    radiotherapy 52–5, 110
    screening (smear test) 24
chemotherapy 12–13, 56–62, 98,
        178, 203–4
    drug resistance 57–8
    route 58–9
    side effects
        bone marrow 60
        diarrhoea 60
        fertility 60–1
        hair loss 59–60
        nausea, vomiting 59
    see also specific organs, regions and
        cancers
Chernobyl Nuclear Reactor 18
childhood tumours 195
cholecystogram 37
chondrosarcoma 161
cigarette smoke *see* smoking
CIN (cervical intraepithelial neoplasia)
        106
cirrhosis 140
cisplatinum 103, 158
clustering of cancers 17–19
colon
    screening 25
    see also bowel
colonoscopy 42
colostomy 130–1
colposcopy 108–9
complementary therapy 205–6, 219–30
computed tomography scanning (CT) 38
contraceptive pill 89–90, 112
counselling 206–7, 222–3
craniopharyngiomas 79
Cushing's syndrome 144
cyclophosphamide, methotrexate and
        5-fluorouracil (CMF) 98

cystoscopy 42, 149
cytotoxic drugs *see* chemotherapy

death and dying 217–18
diagnostic procedures 44
diarrhoea, side effects of chemotherapy
        60
dietary change 228–9
dietary factors 121
    fats 90, 127
DNA 2–4
drinking 140
drugs
    painkillers 210–11
    resistance 57–8
    see also chemotherapy
duodenoscopy 41–2
dysgerminomas 104

eating problems 212–13
emotional support 206–7, 221–3
endometrial cancer 112
endometrium 112
endorphins 212
endoscopy 41–2
environmental factors 17
epidemiology, defined 15–16
epididymitis 156
Epstein–Barr virus 173
ERCP 136
Ewing's sarcoma 160
eye 74–5

faecal occult blood tests 25, 128
fallopian tube carcinoma 105
fats, dietary 90, 127
fertility
    female 60–1, 179
    male 159, 179
    side effects of chemotherapy 60–1
fibre-optics 41–2
fibrosarcoma 165
fistula 155
5-fluorouracil 98, 132–3

function, alteration/loss 30–1

gastrectomy 123
gastroscopy 41–2
genetic factors 90
   familial 19–20
genital wart virus 24
germ cell tumours 104
gliomas 78–82
granulosa cell tumours 105

haemochromatosis 140
haemophoresis 65
hair loss
   chemotherapy 59–60
   radiotherapy 54
head and neck cancers 69–82
   radiotherapy 54
healing therapy 227–8
Helicobacter infection 125
hepatitis 140
hepatoma 140
beta-HGC 35, 156
5-HIAA 35, 139
histiocytoma 161, 165
history of cancer 7–13
Hodgkin's disease 173–84
   bone marrow transplantation 67
hormone levels 87, 97–8, 100
hormone replacement therapy 109, 111
hormone therapy 97–8
hospice care 218
human papillomavirus 5, 107, 155
hypercalcaemia 161
hypothalamus, hormones 98
hysterectomy 102–3, 109–10, 114

immunotherapy 13, 62–8
   see also specific organs, regions and
      cancers
incidence, defined 15–16
indigestion 122
information 215–16
insulin-producing tumours 139

interferons 13, 148, 171–2
interleukin 171
intravenous urogram/pyelogram (IVU)
   38, 109, 149–50
investigations, principles 33–42
iodine, radioactive 76–7
irradiation, total body 49
islet cell tumours 139
itching 214

jaundice 141

kidney 146–9

large cell carcinoma 85
larynx 70
leiomyosarcoma 125, 165
leukaemia 17–19, 30, 187–95
   acute lymphoblastic 187–91
   acute myeloblastic 187–91
   acute myeloid 193
   chronic granulocytic 192–3
   chronic lymphocytic 191, 193–4
   hairy cell 194–5
   multiple myeloma 184–7
   see also bone marrow transplantation
LHRH analogues 98, 115
   pituitary downregulators 98, 115
limb, function loss 31
lip 70
liposarcoma 165
liver 30, 137, 140–3
liver fluke 140
liver function tests 35–6
lung cancer 82–8
   passive smoking 82–3
lymphangiogram 37–8
lymphoedema 214
lymphomas 72, 173
   Burkitt's lymphoma 180
   Hodgkin's disease 67, 173–80
   MALT 125
   non-Hodgkin's lymphoma 67,
      125, 180–4

staging 176
T cell lymphoma 173

magnetic resonance imaging (MRI) 40
male breast cancer 100
malignant fibrous histiocytoma 161, 165
malignant melanoma 167–72
MALT lymphomas 125
mammalian cells 2–4
mammography, screening 23
massage 225–7
mediastinum 160
meditation therapy 227
medulloblastomas 79
melaena stool 32
melanoma 167–72
meningioma 79
menopause
  early 103
  oestrogen reduction 97–8
menstruation 89
mesothelioma 87–8
meta-iodobenzyguanidine (MIBG) 41, 145
metastases 5–6
methotrexate (CMF) 98
mixed mesodermal (mullerian) tumours
    105, 116
moles 168–9
morbidity, defined 15–16
mortality
  coping with dying 217–18
  defined 15–16
  percentages 17
mouth 70
mullerian tumours 105, 116
multiple endocrine neoplasia (MEN) 75
multiple myeloma 184–7
mutations 4
mycosis fungoides 172

naphthylamine 149
nausea
  anti-emetics 213
  side effects of chemotherapy 59
nephroblastoma 146, 197–8

nerve blocks 212
neuroblastoma 144, 195–7
neuroendocrine tumours 139
neurofibrosarcoma 165
nitrates 121
non-Hodgkin's lymphomas 125, 180–4
  bone marrow transplantation 67
nuclear explosions 18
nuclear medicine 41

oat cell carcinoma 85
obstruction 28–9
oesophagoscopy 41–2
oestrogen 97
oncology, defined 7
orchidectomy 100
osteogenic sarcoma 160
ovarian cancer 24–5, 100–5
ovary, screening 24–5

Paget's disease 99–100, 161
pain 29–30, 210–12
painkillers 210–11
palliation 49, 202, 204
  surgery 45–6
pancreas 134–40
papilloma virus (HPV) 5, 107, 155
penis 131, 155
pernicious anaemia 121
phaeochromocytoma 144, 145
Philadelphia chromosome 192
phototherapy 172
pituitary downregulators, LHRH
    analogues 98, 115
platelet transfusions 65–6
platinum drugs 103, 158
polyps, adenomatous polyposis 127
pre-cancerous state 5, 106
prevalence, defined 15–16
progesterone 97, 112, 148
prostate enlargement 151–5
psychotherapy 206–7

quality of life 201–8